10/14 Fit & Smoothie Cleanse

"Unleash the Empowerment to Change Your Lifestyle"

Vickie H. Benson, Ed. D.

Cover Design Photo: Canva

ISBN-13:978-1539598077
ISBN-10:1539598071

Welcome Message

About A Healthier You

Important Disclaimer

Introduction

10/14 Fit & Smoothie Cleanse
"Unleash the Empowerment to Change Your Lifestyle"
Welcome to A Healthier You w/Dr. V. Benson

Thank you for buying this book! I am excited to know that your weight loss journey long awaits you. Losing weight is not easy and being on "Yoyo" diets that have failed you time and time again has brought you to this point. You now have the mind set to do this and I know that you can. I am willing to support and guide you through this transformation. My prayer is that you give God a chance to work this miracle in your life and you trust in Him that He will.

Detoxing and cleansing is needed for everyday health to rejuvenate, increase energy, lose weight, and a jump start to eating healthy foods. Losing weight is not hard. It's only hard to lose weight when your goals are not in focus to maintain the weight lost.

I hope that in reading this book it will help you in planning healthy meals to focus on your desired goals for weight loss. Because I am an effective research-based, science educator, I am adept in providing you with validated, researched information about being healthy. I have spent countless hours reviewing and testing many delicious smoothies, herbal teas, and meal recipes to help with your weight loss. As you meditate and pray daily, invite the Lord, Jesus Christ into your weight loss endeavor to help you stay focused. *"Trust in the Lord with all your heart and lean not to your own understanding, in all your ways acknowledge Him and he will direct your path"* (Proverbs 3:5-6). Now are you ready to take this journey? Let's get started…

A HEALTHIER YOU W/DR.V. BENSON

A Healthier You is a unique detox and cleanse wellness program designed to teach you how to eat healthy and detox the body daily with smoothies, herbal teas, healthy snacks, and meal plans: live well by gaining clarity, vitality, and serenity. This successful detox plan program exceeds beyond expectations because it includes various ways to detox your body even when you are not trying to lose weight.

"A Healthier You" detox and cleanse program will help you to incorporate and manage your eating habits to address many concerns that you may have about healthy living. "A Healthier You" Six-Tier plans have various options on healthy eating that will help you to detox and cleanse the body. The Six-Tier plan includes the 10/14 Fit & Smoothie Cleanse, The Ultimate Healing Foods Plan, 14 Day Detox and Cleanse Plan, Start Eating 5 Day Meal Plan, 7-Day Allergy Detox and Cleanse, and Detox Life After Maintenance Plan.

"A Healthier You" Six Tier plans are not used to diagnosis any chronic illnesses or disorders, but will help you build a program that

is affordable and durable to gain optimal wellness for your chronic illness or disorder. Personal coaching and group coaching is available via my website. Also, you will have access to detox and cleanse plans once you subscribe to the website. When you become VIP member with "A Healthier You", you will receive several perks such as discounts for conferences, online store purchases, healthy eating management plans, coaching, and free recipes.

IMPORTANT DISCLAIMER

***The information printed in this book is for educational usage and has been researched and obtained from various sources.

***I have taught in many areas of Science for nineteen years and have worked in the medical field as a Medical Assistant and Laboratory Technician.

***I am not qualified as a medical provider and information that is written in this book is not to be used for treatment or cure for any health conditions.

***I am not licensed as a medical provider to diagnose, treat or cure any medical condition or advise on the condition. I do not provide other services that aids in medical or psychological advice.

***Consult with your medical healthcare provider before deciding to use any of the detox plans if you are unsure about changing your diet, adding supplements, or using any nutritional recipe plans.

***Use sound judgement if you decide to use any of the recipes or plans I have written and consult with your healthcare provider. If any of the recipes contain foods that you are allergic to, **avoid** the food item in the recipe. Once again consult with your healthcare provider for advice.

INTRODUCTION

There are hundreds of books, nutritionist, weight loss clinics, counselors, diet programs, health coaches, and many other resources available that defines the best way to detox and cleanse our bodies. The resources are very legitimate in providing such relevant information. In fact, this is how I got started with learning how to detox and cleanse my body. I felt the need to write, develop, and incorporate my own plan that is very beneficial in relating to those who have chronic illnesses such as hypertension, diabetes, and high cholesterol, especially for educators and those who work 9 to 5. Many people are experiencing problems with weight gain, fatigue/low energy or no energy, bloating, PMS, anxiety, headaches, memory loss, infections, excess swelling of the feet and hands, allergy problems, and other illnesses.

There is no one miracle magical spell for weight loss, but I tell you the best weight loss plan has been here, right before our eyes for decades. It is natural and healthy for our bodies to maintain optimal health. Everything about eating healthy, and thriving to be healthy, is good.

I struggled with my weight for many years. I have been on so many diets, like the cabbage soup diet, 3-day high protein diet, low-carb diet (Adkins), and have even taken diet and water pills. You name it, I have done it. Little did I know that just a simple detox and cleanse would be the answer... I would have done this a long time ago. Now that God has given me spiritual growth and insight on how to help myself and others to heal the body through detox and cleansing, I am excited to do that just for you. ***"Do not be wise in your own eyes; fear the Lord and shun evil. This will bring health to your body and nourishment to your bones" (Proverbs 3:7-8).***

Chapter 1

MY STORY

I have taught in the education system for nearly 19 years. Teaching in many areas of science and in combination of being a successful leader, coach, and researcher, there had to be something else I could do with my educational degrees besides teaching in the classroom. I wanted a new perspective on life. I needed to change my inner being so that I could make a difference in the way that I looked and felt about my weight.

You see, I have had many illnesses my entire life. At age 7, scarlet fever changed my skin color two shades darker. Healing from the scarlet fever, I started having seizures, took phenobarbital for 6 years, and the seizures stopped at age 10.

The years past and my weight increased, my feet and hands were always swelling, I was anemic, I had many sinus infections, occasional strep throat, and took allergy shots yearly avoid being ill. In 1993, I was faced with emergency gallstone surgery and my gall bladder was removed. Gastroenteritis was intolerable and was hospitalized several times due inflammation. I recall having a 24-hour stomach virus and drove to the hospital in excruciating pain. Not knowing that my body was full of toxins and my white blood cells were working hard to fight off the infection due to processed food that I had eaten from a local restaurant.

In year 2000, I was diagnosed with an infected fallopian tube that was surgically removed along with a myomectomy due to numerous fibroids. One fibroid was the size of a grapefruit that protruded the lumbar and resulted in Chiropractic therapy. With excessive bloating and bleeding during my cycle, with a uterus the size of a 6-month old pregnant woman, feet swelling and hanging over my shoes, and wanted to have another child past the age of 40, I lost all hope to be happy and healthy. I didn't feel good about myself. I was miserable and resulted to unhealthy food for comfort. That is when the weight started to pile on.

My fibroids had grown back after nearly one year. Faced with the option of having a hysterectomy, I decided not to go that route because of previous surgeries. So, I had a second myomectomy due to the growth of the fibroids in 2002. The surgery was unsuccessful because of excessive scare tissue. However, the fibroids continued to give me problems and I developed hormonal issues, especially with acne breakouts.

I really didn't understand at my age, why I had bad acne problems. I sought two different dermatologists, bought several topical cleansers, took tetracycline (antibiotic to help with acne), changed makeup several times, and stop drinking sodas for a while. I did increase my water intake, but still loved juice that was loaded with refined sugar.

In 2011, embolization was the new radiologic invasive procedure to eliminate fibroids. I decided to go through the procedure because the recovery time was short. Recovery from the embolization was very painful for several days. My blood pressure was out of control after the procedure because of the pain medication, however, that was the only time my blood pressure had spiked 200/140, normal blood pressure 120/80. But thank God I recovered. In 2012, I had an ablation procedure due to excessive bleeding 1 year later from the embolization. I had believed the ablation was the miracle I had looked for, but soon had other complications from the ablation procedure.

In the Summer of 2013, while I was in job transition, I decided to do something about my weight, but before I could get things going, an unexpected allergic reaction invaded my body and several allergy shots followed. When antibodies are triggered due to an allergic reaction, that is a sign that toxins are invading the body. Even when your skin is often itchy, dry or the skin feels crawly, that is also a sign of toxins invading the body. Eventually the white blood cells fight to get rid of foreign invaders and the allergic reaction subside until the next go round.

Upon healing from the allergic attack, I refocused and decided to do something about my weight again. I ordered a NutriBullet from an infomercial that I had seen on TV on numerous occasions. While watching the infomercial, I noticed how vegetables and fruits were blended to revert many health issues. People were seeing results in as little as 3 to 4 days. As a science teacher, I knew that when food is blended, it could be broken down to extract the nucleus, but didn't think that the nutrients from the food were beneficial to the body afterwards.

Once I received my NutriBullet, I started making tasty green smoothies. Never thought fruit and vegetables blended could taste so good. My energy level was enormously shooting through the roof, I was sleeping better, my though process was in focus, and I dropped 30 pounds in one month. Just by drinking green smoothies.

So, I continued drinking the green smoothies and started an aerobics routine using Leslie Sansone "Walk-A-Way the Pounds" video, taking long walks in the neighborhood, and even going to the gym where I lived. I lost another astounding 10 lbs. I thought had everything under control. My job transition was looking good, I was moving to a new state with a clear mindset, my energy level was great, and I was happy with my weight loss.

By November 2013, I gained over half of the pounds back. Some of my health issues returned. Many allergy infections, headaches, postnasal drip, strep throat, poor sleep pattern, fatigue, stress, and weight gain. A reoccurrence of upper respiratory problems returned for what I thought was long gone. I had returned to my old eating habits and literally stop exercising. I have always been active. I marched in the band from high school to college and have never had a problem with exercising.

I realized for me to be healthy, I had to commit and make a major decision to eliminate foods that I did not need such as processed can, fried, and fast foods, including cakes, pies, cookies, ice cream, potato chips, candy, pizza, spaghetti, donuts, and pasta. You name it, I ate it. I drunk diet sodas, sweet tea, lemonade and juice loaded with sugar, occasional wine, and very little water. Soon afterwards, I started having hot flashes and couldn't tolerate the heat nor the cold sweats. I thought I was losing it. My body was really toxic at this point, but I didn't know it.

My attitude was like a fire ball. My health was declining and I added about 20 more lbs to what I had lost during the Summer. I needed to find some stability, clarity, serenity, and motivation to get healthy and stay healthy. I may have gained 15 more pounds and reached a whopping 270 lbs within a 2-year span. I was disengaged and needed help to get the weight off. I could not see myself reaching 300 lbs.

In 2015, I made a pledge to be healthier before I turned 50. If I would have kept going the way that I was, I probably would have ended up with a very serious chronic illness such as diabetes or hypertension. Diabetes and hypertension reached back as far as my grandmother and several of my family members. I didn't want to encounter being burden with taken medication. So, I prayed and asked God to help me with my weight. I still pray daily about my weight; I never want to go back to unhealthy eating again.

I begin to research for healthy diets and came across JJ. Smith's *"10 Day Green Smoothie"* book. In fact, I stumbled upon her Facebook page and ordered the book. Little did I know the day I decided to start on the "10 Day Green Smoothie" cleanse, was the day JJ. Smith challenged millions on her Facebook group page to start the *"10 Day Green Smoothie Challenge"*. My sister Rhonda told me about the challenge, but it was conformation in the spirit that God was leading me in this direction. How ironic for me to start with others across the world who was on the same path to losing weight in a healthy way.

By my 50th birthday, I was down 18lbs. I took in 10 days of green smoothies, ate healthy, snacks, rested, and did no exercises. For 10 whole days, I did this. Who would have thought this could happened so fast, again? Losing weight that is. When I think back on how I was drinking the green smoothies in 2013 and losing weight, I didn't realize how the green smoothies played such an amazing factor for keeping me healthy. My skin was clear, my thoughts were clear, I slept better, and my energy level was awesome once again. My body was overloaded with toxins and this kept me ill and over weight for years. To be honest, I didn't know that toxins were the problem or that parasites could invade the body to cause chronic illnesses. I knew that parasites could enter the body to do harm, but not to cause symptoms that leads to illnesses such as:

> "diabetes, hypertension, migraines, gas bloating, belly fat, excess weight, vision problems, back pain, constipation/diarrhea, Bruxism, post nasal drip, allergies, nasal itching, joint pain, digestive disorders, anemia, prostatitis, muscle cramps, skin problems, irritable bowel syndrome, craving *(clay, dirt, raw rice, dried foods, charcoal, pasta, burned foods)* disturbed sleep *(night sweats, fatigue, crawling sensations),* headaches, poor blood circulation, weakness, pain around the eyes, bruising, bad breath, and foot fungus".

These are only a few of the symptoms listed about how parasites invade our bodies to cause illness. Doctor's don't tell us about parasites and problems they may cause within the body. We go from day to day not knowing that processed foods cause abnormalities that we cannot see, but feel. Therefore, we believe it to be normal, but it is not. God gets the glory for giving JJ. Smith's *"10 Day Green Smoothie Challenge"* life. The challenge put me back on the right path and inspired me to be "A Healthier Me"! ***Where there's no vision the people will perish" (Proverbs 29:18).***

I changed my eating habits, within 6 months I lost 56 lbs, in 10 months 62 lbs, and holding steady. It was more than exciting to see such a tremendous weight loss just by eating healthy planned meals, healthy snacks, and making delicious smoothies to replace 2 and sometimes 3 meals a day. Smoothies are so powerful, enriched with antioxidants, and vitamins that I no longer take multivitamins. The only supplement I take daily is coconut oil 1000 mg per day. A miracle in its self. I truly needed to be strong and healthy. My prayers were answered and I have continued the path to eating healthy.

Some people have asked me, "Have you ever gotten off track while trying to eat healthy foods or have been in plateau?" Of course, I have gotten off track and have plateaued, but have learned that, even if I got off track, I always regained focus to do the right thing. I may have eaten a bowl of vanilla ice cream with fudge and caramel syrup or a bag of cheddar cheese potato chips with chocolate chip cookies, but I detox daily to maintain, even if I slip up. You won't gain weight in one day just because you were tempted to eat the wrong foods. As far as plateauing, all it takes is a few minor changes to make it work back in your favor. Adding more protein to the diet to burn the fat, drink more water, smoothies if necessary (more greens), lemon water, and/or herbal tea to push the bowels out or the body, more sleep and exercise. Know what your body need to move the fat once you have gone overboard in eating the wrong foods.

I have been more than just motivated to have developed "A Healthier You" Detoxify and Cleanse program. The program has allowed me to know who I am and what I can do to help others to be healthy. I am determined to get as many people to look at healthy eating as a blessing from God. It is in the food that God has given us to heal the body. *"Worship the Lord your God, and His blessings will be on your food and water. I will take away sickness among you"* (Exodus 23:25).

With smoothies, herbal detox teas, meal plans, and healthy snacks, it will change your way of looking at food in a different way. Eating healthy keeps your body free from toxins that causes chronic illnesses, inflammation, and many disease-causing disorders. These unwanted illnesses are so vulnerable and are capable for making the body homeostatic imbalanced.

Eating healthy ensures clarity, vitality, and serenity which is the key to a better way of life and wellness. I hope that you have decided to dedicate a life time of good clean eating to become a "A healthier You"! I hope you will join the revolution and continue this journey with me. I will be detoxing and cleansing every day and want you to do the same!

Chapter 2

DETOX and CLEANSE QUESTIONNAIRE

Are you eating processed foods such as lunching meats, canned foods, frozen TV foods? Do you crave for sugar (sweets), carbohydrates, and or eat pasta all the time? Do you drink more than 1 cup of coffee per day, crave other caffeinated beverages or drink performance enhancement products to rev-up your metabolism? Are you gaining weight while snacking on cookies, potato chips, donuts, or candy? Do you often eat fried foods, fast foods, or eat late at night? If all these things are causing you to gain weight, lack energy and sleep, have skin problems (acne, oily, scaly or dry), have memory fog, or feeling fatigue, then it is possible you need to detox and cleanse your body to eliminate parasites that are invaders that thrive in unhealthy bodies. Do you want to win your clarity, vitality and serenity back from these nasty parasites? You can with the *10/14 Fit & Smoothie Cleanse.*

I have created a questionnaire for you. Take the time to rate the symptoms that you typically are having to determine if you need a detox due to health issues and poor eating habits. Use the point scale below to complete the questionnaire. Total your points and see what the results are to determine your needs.

Point Scale:

0 – I don't need a detox, but you have concerns about other health issues.

1 – I occasionally have these symptoms, but they are not severe and I probably could use a detox.

2 – I occasionally have these symptoms, but they are slight severe and I probably could use a detox.

3 – I frequently have these symptoms, and I can use a detox.

4 – I frequently have these symptoms, but they are severe and I can use a detox.

Symptoms	Points
Headaches/Migraines/Dizziness	
Bloating/Indigestion/Frequent gas after eating	
Lack of Sleep/Insomnia	
Colds or flu like symptoms	
Allergies	
Brain Fog/Memory Loss	
Fatigue/Tired/Drowsiness/Sluggish/Lack of Energy	
Drink coffee or any caffeine products daily	
Chemical sensitivity	
Constipation/ Less than one bowel movement per day.	
Joint pain	
Sugar cravings or Carb Cravings	
Weight gain	
Poor concentration	
Mood swing	
Anger/Irritability/Aggressiveness	

Depression/Sad	
Acne/Pimples/Blemishes Rashes/Hives	
Reoccurring Sinus Infections/Postnasal Drip/ Congestion/Ear Infections	
Bags/Dark circles under the eyes	
Hot flashes	
Impotence	
Water retention	
Exposed environmental toxins (Car exhaustion/factors	
Hypertension	
Diabetes	
Bad Breath/Coated tongue, gums, and lips/Decaying of the Teeth	
Blurred vision/Itchy and burning eyes	
Itchy or Dry Skin	
Acid Reflux	
Stress/Anxiety/Antsy	
Total Score	

Results

> ➤ If you scored **25 or higher**, you can benefit from a detox and cleanse. It will help with weight loss, boost your energy level, and possibly revert some chronic illnesses.

> ➤ If you scored between *10 and 20*, you are more than likely can benefit from one of the A Healthier You 6Tier Plans.

> ➤ If you scored *5 or below*, you may not need a detox and very little intervention is needed for a clean bill of health. Just a few minor changes in your eating habits.

Chapter 3

WHY SHOULD I DETOX?

Our bodies are self-cleansers, but unfortunately it doesn't always work in our favor. The body is just like Spring cleaning. Spring is a time for new beginnings. The body needs a Spring cleaning to function properly. Our body works hard daily to cleanse the waste and toxins that embeds its self in our cells. In most cases, our body can't effectively thoroughly cleanse because we don't eat the right foods.

Although our bodies are self-cleansers, it can only clean-up a few cells to get rid of the toxins. These toxins affect our metabolism, behavior, and immune system that leads to diseases. When our body is overloaded with toxins, it breaks down, and it can't handle the changes that toxins causes, especially when we are not eating the right foods to stay healthy. Once the body breaks down from consuming the wrong foods, that is when sickness and disease occur. Everybody can benefit from a detox and cleanse. Not just to lose weight, but to stay healthy.

The waste that we consume invades our body and comes from food that is undigested or by-products of natural metabolic processes such as:

- Environmental factors (Polluted air from near-by factories, car exhaustion, airborne viruses, cancer-causing chemicals, preservatives, pesticides, heavy metals, and industrial waste)
- Contagious diseases and infections (Bacterium and viruses)
- Chemicals (Household products and body fragrances)

Our bodies are made in the image and likeness of God. We must take care of our body just like He does. When the body is unstable it is *Dis-Eased* which is homeostatic imbalanced. Our bodies are meant to be homeostasis, a stable internal environment. We create most of our sickness due to our eating habits. However, the body deteriorates due to the lack of eating proper nutrients while other toxins sneak into the body that decrease our wellness causing degenerative diseases that surges within us daily.

If we are eating healthy and doing it consistently, our unhealthy issues will keep us out of the doctor's office and will help decrease healthcare cost. We must cleanse and detoxify our bodies frequently and make choices that will benefit us for a life time. Let's make changes where they are mostly needed to promote a clean bill of health as well as teach others to do the same. Remember this is a lifestyle change not a diet. You will love to be "A Healthier You" of wellness through detoxing and cleansing.

Chapter 4

PREPARING FOR THE CLEANSE

Let's say you prepare for 25 people to come over for a dinner party. You prep the food to make sure you have enough for at least 2 to 3 servings per guest. When the dinner party is over, you clean the kitchen and throw away trash after the guest leaves, but have leftovers that you may eat for the next day or two. Leftover food can build on more toxins in the body that is not eliminated through proper cleansing.

Detoxing and cleansing, allows you to get rid of the leftovers that can later cause you to gain weight. You have leftovers that you don't need in your body too, such as extra fat, excessive bloating, aches and pain. This is due to the body consuming and eating unhealthy foods. However, when you prep for the cleanse, be sure to follow the exact smoothie recipes to receive your daily nutrients, including water to take the leftovers out of the body.

Prepping your food during the cleanse is so important. You save time with prepping your food, especially if you work early mornings or late nights. You save money too, by freezing your leafy greens to keep them from ruining. Buying leafy greens can be expensive. If you prep all your meals daily, you will eat healthy foods throughout the day and become more excited about your results as you move through the cleanse.

If you don't like water, I want you to understand that water is the key to helping in detoxification. Our bodies are made up of 60% to 80% of water and it is needed for hydration, to make our skin supple and keeps it from drying out, cushions our organs, flushes out body fat and keeps the fat away. To make water taste better just add lemon. But make sure that you get in half your body weight of water daily. For example, if you weigh 140 lbs you will drink approximately 4 ½ ozs of bottled water which equals 16.9 fl. ozs.

Leaping into this journey, you will learn how committed you are in maintaining your health. This is a new chapter in your life and progressing forward will be beneficial to you. Personal support will be provided to help you through this process so that you will be able to finish strong.

What happens if you fall off a wagon? You get up and get back on the wagon. Just like detoxing, you may get off track, but don't be defeated, move on to the next day and continue with the 10/14 Fit & Smoothie Cleanse. Many people have detoxed and derailed, even I have, especially when I have cooked a full course delicious meal for my family. I derail dangerously. The aroma and richness of the food is so amazing, that I have to eat it too. I would fix myself a small plate to eat my delicious food and enjoy every minute. I felt guilty and good at the same time, because I might have had seconds. However, I would jump back on track the next day without derailing again, because I knew what my goals were. It is okay to pick up where you left off, but don't let it get too far. You don't want to lose hope of getting healthy. So, fight hard to stay focus!

Now is the time to make that serious commitment and jump start your healthy lifestyle. Get on track from where you are now! Start prepping for the "10/14" today. Don't worry about "Can I do this?" "Is detoxing for me?", "Am I going to starve?", "What will my friends say?", "Will my family support me?" These questions have been thought provoking before from many people, even me. Keep the goal in mind that you want a healthy lifestyle. You have made the commitment to eating healthy and taking control of any drastic changes in your life that has kept you from eating the right foods. Don't worry, you will do fine. God got you in this!

Explore your options about your health. Do you want to be vibrant, strong, and healthy or do you want to sit and wait for the weight to continue to pile on? You must step back and make whatever changes that are needed for a life time to gain adequate results. Of course, you will not see a fast change, but I guarantee you that you will see and feel a necessary change that is much needed for a healthy body. Although change is gradually done during the cleansing process for the body, it will allow the body to repair itself naturally inside and out. Even with stretching the body, avoiding refine sugars, gluten, and process products will eliminate toxins and repair the body for wellness.

To get things under control, you must start cleaning your house. You know if your house has things laying around you must pick them up and put it in its proper place. To prepare for the cleanse your refrigerator will no longer need all the foods that have kept you from eating healthy. This includes cleaning out your food pantry too! I can recall, the only thing I needed out of my food pantry during the cleanse were my raw nuts and seeds. Once you get the items you need for the cleanse, your refrigerator would resemble the nicely neat veggie and fruit stands that we see in are local food stores or at a farmer's market.

So, I guess a refrigerator cleaning is needed to clear out everything that is unhealthy before the detoxing and cleansing starts. This doesn't mean you can't freeze some of the items for after the cleanse. I know in the back of your mind you are wondering how in the world am I going to get rid of the cookies, potato chips, and candy in my pantry before the cleanse. Well, you don't! Just look at it this way, resistance is needed, but if you have made that serious commitment and you start the cleanse right, you will not have an urgency to eat what is in the pantry that caused you to have headaches, diabetes, hypertension, extra belly fat, and excess weight. Therefore, you should detox and cleanse daily to eliminate the toxins from your life forever.

Don't keep struggling with an intoxicated body. Cleanse, for a renewing of your strength, clarity, vitality, and serenity.

1 Corinthians 6:19 says *"Don't you realize that your body is the temple of the Holy Spirit, who lives in you and was given to you by God? You do not belong to yourself"*. Pray for God's temple to be cleansed with the renewing of your mind. We are a part of God's body. He wants us to live strong, happy, and healthy.

Chapter 5

LET THE CLEANSING PROCESS BEGIN

This is your challenge! Let's get to it. On day one you will encounter the "I can't do this syndrome", "it's too hard", and "I am hungry". Around 12 noon you smell every food scent that entices your hunger pain and you want it and you may buy it. **DON'T** do it! Let me tell you, it is possible to revert from clean healthy eating from morning to unhealthy eating at noon. This is typical for someone who has never detoxed and cleanse before. The strategy is to avoid foods that adds on unwanted fat, but eat foods that substrates the fat from the body. Mind over matter is the key to wanting a healthy lifestyle.

If this is not your first cleanse and you didn't make it through the first day, I hope that you will start on day 2. Regain focus and pull through the snares of beginner's detox and cleanse. Write, type or take a picture of these tips below. Place the tips on your refrigerator and food pantry door as reminders in hope to keep you strong.

Simple tips to get you through your very first detox and cleanse:

AHY TIP 1: Pray and meditate to ask for strength for the cleanse, the ability to eliminate all uninvited toxins, parasites, and unwanted illnesses from the body.

AHY TIP 2: Before starting a cleanse, you want to drink room temperature bottled water with squeezed lemon or lemon juice. Hydrating with the lemon water is essential for preparing the body for the cleanse and you will get an early start for detoxing the liver and kidney.

AHY Tip 3: Drink herbal detox tea the night before. The teas I suggest are Super Dieter's Tea, Smoothe Move, or Hyleys Detox or Slim Tea to get rid of fecal material from the day before. However, if you work in the mornings, don't bother drinking the tea the night before because you may be occupying the restroom all day. It is okay to skip this step because you will be using this process during the cleanse, but do drink the squeezed lemon or lemon juice water if you don't drink the herbal teas the night before.

AHY Tip 4: Drink more water or lemon water, at least to prepare to hydrate the body to avoid headaches and irritability for any withdrawal reaction when the cleanse starts. If you drink caffeinated coffee or soda's daily, **STOP!** This will help to eliminate some symptoms while on the cleanse if you reframe from daily intake of caffeinated beverages. Symptoms include severe to moderate headaches, nausea, insomnia, and irritability. Remember to use the water to body weight ratio to help decrease the symptoms. Symptoms will disappear within a few days.

AHY Tip 5: Evaluate your food list and get exactly what is on the list to make this a very successful cleanse and detox. Follow the 10/14 Fit & Smoothie Cleanse plan as written to avoid any hiccups. If you do have hiccups, just continue to the next day. Stay encourage and remember you are not on a DIET!

During the cleanse, you must eliminate refine sugars, breads, flour, saturated fats, processed foods, preservatives, artificial colors and chemical foods. Foods that contain these substances keeps us fat, bloated, tired, irritable, and invades our bodies with diseases, infections, and overloads the body with toxins. Our organs try to keep up with what the function of the body is supposed to do once it is invaded with toxins, but it can't, because it is trying so hard to get rid of the bad stuff just so it can live.

Chapter 6

10/14 GROCERY LIST

ORGANIC FOODS vs. NATURAL FRESH FOODS

Your 10/14 grocery list is divided into two weeks to prevent spoilage. Check off as you buy to avoid buying twice the amount of food. Buy organic when you can, but fresh natural food is good too. However, some experts believe that organic foods are free of preservatives, pesticides, and herbicides. Organic foods are monitored by the government. While fresh and natural foods are synthesized, and are not monitored by the government. When choosing natural foods, examine the quality, wash, and store in the freezer to avoid spoilage.

Although there is no sound evidence of organic foods being healthier than fresh natural foods, it is the thought of knowing that organic foods are monitored and has a longer shelve life. Recent research suggests choosing organic foods can increase heavy antioxidants and eliminate heavy toxin metals. On the other hand, others feel that processing organic foods can disturb the health benefits and prefer to choose natural foods.

GROCERY LIST

	Week One	
Size	**Grocery Items**	**Check**
20 oz.	Spinach	
20 oz.	Kale	
20 oz.	Spring Mix Greens	
1 Bag	Celery Stalks	
1 1b or 1-6.75 oz.	Ginger Root Grounded Ginger	
1 Bag	Flaxseeds (Grounded or Milled)	
1 Box	Stevia	
1 Box	Stevia	
1 Bag or Jar	Sunflower Seeds (Unsalted)	
1 Case or 4 Gallons	Purified or Distilled Water	
16 oz.	Frozen or Fresh Blueberries	
16 oz.	Frozen Strawberries	
16 oz.	Frozen Pineapple Chunks	
16. oz.	Frozen Mango	
16 oz.	Frozen Mixed Berries	
1 Bag	Green Apples	
1 Box	Stevia	
1 Bag or Jar	Sunflower Seeds (Unsalted)	
1 Case or 4 Gallons	Purified or Distilled Water	
16 oz.	Frozen or Fresh Blueberries	
16 oz.	Frozen Strawberries	
16 oz.	Frozen Pineapple Chunks	
16. oz.	Frozen Mango	
16 oz.	Frozen Mixed Berries	
1 Bag	Green Apples	
1	Cucumber	
1	Lime	
1	Kiwi	
5	Bananas	
1	Orange	
½ lb.	Green Seedless Grapes	
32 oz. or 1 Bag	100% Pure Lemon Juice or Lemons	
	Non-Dairy Plant Based Protein Powder; Organic Purely Inspired or Raw Protein by Garden Life or Sun Warrior Protein	
Snacks	Fruit and Veggies of Choice (Carrots, Celery, Green Apples)	
Snacks	Raw or Unsalted Nuts and Seeds	

	Yogi Detox Tea or Hyley's Wellness Detox Tea or Traditional Medicinal Everyday Detox Tea	
	Decaffeinated Lipton Green Tea Pomegranate	
	Yogi Skin Detox Tea and/or Cinnamon Vanilla Healthy Skin Tea	
	Life Style Awareness Hibiscus Cleanse	
1 Box	Epsom Salt with or without Menthol (Feet Detox)	
1 Bottle	Mag 07 **(OPTIONAL)** Used for bowel movement	
1 Box	Unionized Salt **(OPTIONAL)** If you are not hypertensive you may purchase) for Salt Water Flush (SWF)	
	Yogi Detox Tea or Hyleys Wellness Detox Tea, Traditional Medicinal Everyday Detox Tea or Yogi Smoothe Move	
	Week Two	
Size	**Grocery Item**	**Check**
20 oz.	Spinach	
20 oz.	Kale	
20 oz.	Spring Mix Greens	
1 Bag	Celery Stalks	
1 lb	Ginger Root or 1- 6.75 oz. Grounded Ginger	
1 Bag	Flaxseeds (Grounded or Milled)	
1 Case or 4 Gallons	Purified or Distilled Water	
1 Bag	Almonds (Unsalted or Raw)	
1 Bag	Walnuts (Unsalted or Raw)	
2	Bananas	
1 Bag	Green Apples	
2	Cucumbers	
3	Oranges	
2 Bunches	Parsley	
1 Small	Tomato	
16 oz. Bag	Carrots	
16 oz.	Frozen Blueberries	
16 oz.	Frozen Mixed Berries	
16 oz.	Frozen Mixed Mango	
16 oz.	Frozen Pineapple Chunks	
16 oz.	Frozen or Fresh Cranberries	
16 oz.	Frozen Mixed Fruit	
16 oz.	Frozen or Fresh Blackberries	

½ lb.	Red Seedless Grapes	
½ lb.	Green Seedless Grapes	
½ lb.	Black Seedless Grapes (Optional)	
32 oz. or 1 Bag	100 % Lemon Juice or Lemons	
1.25 oz.	Cinnamon	
1.2 oz.	Turmeric	
	Non-Dairy Plant Based Protein Powder; Organic Purely Inspired or Raw Protein by Garden Life or Sun Warrior Protein	
Snacks	Fruit and Veggies of Choice (Carrots, Celery, Green Apples)	
Snacks	Raw or Unsalted Nuts and Seeds	
	Decaffeinated Lipton Green Tea	
	Braggs Apple Cider Vinegar with the mother in the bottle (the brownish settlement at the bottom.	
	Yogi Detox Tea or Hyleys Wellness Detox Tea or Traditional Medicinal Everyday Detox Tea or Yogi Smoothe Move	
	Decaffeinated Lipton Green Tea Pomegranate	
	Yogi Skin Detox Tea and/or Cinnamon Vanilla Healthy Skin Tea	
	Life Style Awareness Hibiscus Cleanse	
1 Bag	Epsom Salt with or without Menthol (Feet Detox)	
1 Bottle	Mag 07	
1 Box	Unionized Salt **(OPTIONAL)** If you are not hypertensive you may purchase) for Salt Water Flush (SWF)	

Note:

You may have enough food items for 10 and 14 days. You will not have to buy additional food based on the grocery list. If you decide to use fresh fruits and veggies, do not wash until you are ready to make smoothies or you can freeze them, but wash before freezing. Fresh veggies and fruit spoil quickly when washed before using.

Chapter 7

EATING EXPENSIVE FOODS

Eating healthy is expensive. But it's all for good health. Now that you are getting ready for the cleanse, if by any chance you can start purchasing organic fruits and vegetables, raw nuts and seeds (unsalted), it would be great. If you cannot purchase organic, fresh fruits and vegetables, the cleanse will work the same. Save time in preparing your smoothies by thoroughly washing the fruit, Ziploc bag them, and store fruit and leafy greens in the freezer until ready to use. I also recommend that you purchase frozen fruit. Frozen fruit provides the thickness, keeps the smoothie cold, and creamer. Try to avoid ice, if possible. Ice waters the smoothie down into a liquid and gives the smoothie a bland taste. Purchase herbal teas, purified or spring water to stay hydrated and to push belly fat. ***See 10/14 grocery list***. Homemade herbal teas have a delicious flavor and helps to fight toxins in the body. Spices are good to add to herbal teas. One spice for sure will boost your metabolism and help with weight loss, is cayenne and ginger. You can add ginger to any of the *"Detox Herbal Teas"* it reduces hunger up to six hours. Cayenne can be added to help with belly fat loss *(see recipe for belly fat with cayenne and apple cider vinegar)*.

Always prep the night before or prep for at least 3 days in advance to avoid the early morning rush, if you work early mornings. I don't want you to leave your lunch and dinner or snacks at home.

If you are like me, and like making smoothies without prepping, go ahead and prep the same day. Avoid washing your leafy veggies and storing them in the refrigerator. They tend to get soggy. Unless you like soggy veggies. Freezing the veggies would be better. Wash the veggies before putting them into the smoothies. Some veggie packages say pre-wash. Still rinse the vegetables for safety precautions. Use medium size Ziploc bags and a permanent marker to write the days on the bags. Store in the refrigerator or freezer until ready to use. Prepping for 5 days at a time is better.

Staying strong during the cleanse can be very difficult, especially if this is the first cleanse. Pre-plan for the cleanse. Give yourself time to read the entire book, go over your grocery list, search for reasonable food prices, and understand the benefits of the detox and cleanse. The more you focus on getting healthier the better you will feel mentally and physically.

Chapter 8

WHAT AM I DOING?

Let's be realistic! You have never done a cleanse before and more than likely you may or may not want to do a cleanse ever again. I felt the same way. When I finally had the mindset to do the detox and cleanse, I thought I was not going to make it through the first day. It was hard! I was having food withdrawal symptoms, headaches, and cravings. However, after 24 hours, and a good night sleep, I felt amazing. I had more energy and my body felt light.

Now that you have examined your symptoms from the self-questionnaire in *Chapter 2*, do you feel that you need a detox and cleanse? Don't think twice about not detoxing and cleansing, especially if you scored 10 or higher on the questionnaire. Everyone can benefit from a cleanse. Some people may not realize that the body is overloaded with toxins that are from the environment and processed foods. These toxins cause chronic illnesses such as diabetes, hypertension, fibromyalgia, arthritis, osteoporosis, high cholesterol, fibroids, impotence, autism, Alzheimer's and other chronic diseases that keep people from having an active healthy lifestyle. Due to toxins, others suffer from weight gain, fatigue, headaches, infections, memory loss, bloating, edema and other troubled symptoms of a toxic body.

Answer these few questions and evaluate your answers. Do you believe that your body needs a cleanse? Really, how clean is your body? Are you having any reoccurrence of the same illness? Clearly if you assessed your health needs based on the few questions in the survey, and your score was10 and above, do you understood that your body may need a thorough cleanse? Have you ever looked at your carpeted floors a week after vacuuming and they look clean to you? If your carpet is not vacuumed at least once a week, it will collect everything from dust to dirt, and to black unwanted spots that can't see. Our bodies do the same thing. The body collects unwanted junk that we put inside of it and accumulates stuff that we didn't need. So, we get frustrated, tired, we have body pains, infections, diabetes, hypertension, low energy, over eat and other problems. Only because we have excess trash/leftovers in our bodies that don't belong in us. Until we do something about it, then the trash/leftovers stays there.

Usually we will get sick eventually if we are not eating right, we take prescribed medication to help with the cure which can cause toxins. We even may have to spend some time in the hospital before we can return back to "good ole' healthy". So, we think it is good health. It is not! That excess trash is still circulating and storing its self in the fat compartments throughout the body daily until we get sick again. Are you in need of a detox and cleanse?

Chapter 9

WHAT IF?

Just imagine always being alert, sleeping well, waking up rejuvenated every morning without enhancers to give the body an energy boost or to stay awake during the day. What if the headaches you've had for the past two weeks or for 5 years where gone? What if you could finally see deflated feet and hands without the swelling or without the pain? Or the stiffness of joints? What if you have less stress and able to think clearly? What if you can get rid of the bloated belly and belly fat, decrease the painful menstrual cycles, have your diabetes under control, lower or eliminate your high blood pressure, revert irritable bowel syndrome, or even gastritis? What if you could get rid all these diseases or disorders that's causing you from being healthy? You can, with a detox and cleanse.

The plan that I have developed will help you to thrive so that you can become healthier, is detoxing and cleansing for body. Detoxing and cleansing does work. I thought, "what if I can help others to achieve the same accomplishments based on the same goals and values that I saw benefitted me after my detoxing and cleansing process"? "What will be the outcome for others"? I had to step out on faith as God directed me to develop a plan that will heal myself and others. In fact, I developed several plans that address many health issues. However, before taking this step, you must agree to change your eating habits and choose the right foods that will make you healthy. Ask yourself these questions. What if I start today? What results will I see? What if this changes my health situation for a life time? What if my chronic illness reverts? The only way you will know these answers to the questions is to start. Once you have achieved your goals, continue with your healthy lifestyle, and set examples that will help others to become healthy too.

Chapter 10

HOW TO DO THE 10/14 FIT & SMOOTHIE CLEANSE

Detoxing with the right foods will nourish the body, mind, and inner spirit. The *10/14 Fit & Smoothie Cleanse* will help you to become healthy while embracing the goodness of healthy eating and enjoy what you are eating. It will change your life forever! It has made me appreciate the value of eating healthy foods. We must be thankful that God has allowed us to take in all His natural fruits and veggies that keeps us thriving. I don't know what I would have done at this point in my life if I would not have been introduced to detoxing and cleansing, and eating healthy daily.

I solely believe that this is the way detoxing and cleansing should be done, eating good healthy wholesome food every day without worrying about inflicted diseases or disorders that may eventually harm the body. However, as I began to examine the makeup of the *10/14 Fit & Smoothie Cleanse,* I focused on specifics for the inner and outer body areas that would help in weight loss and chronic illnesses.

The *10/14 Fit & Smoothie Cleanse* is uniquely designed to cleanse every organ inside of your body including the largest organ of body the "skin". Yes, the skin! If the skin is invaded with any toxins or impurities from the environment, the body will easily become toxic on the inside and outside.

Although the skin is the first line of defense, it can still absorb toxins because of open pores which eventually manifest itself in our blood stream. Then our cells become damage and therefore we get ill. Environmental factors that causes damage to our cells are exposure to chemical toxins (e.g. smoking or second hand smoke, pollution, pesticides, household cleaners, food toxins, toxic metals, or medical x-rays), and infection by some bacteria and viruses (e.g. Flu, colds, Helicobacter Pylori) and, water sources (e.g. tap water, fountain, pools).

Once the body starts to release toxins, the skin glows clearing any imperfections of the skin, especially if you are having skin disorders such as acne, blackheads, oily or dry skin, itchy, psoriasis, and eczema. Taking 1000 mg of coconut oil will help heal the skin also. Coconut oil has an enormous amount of benefits. Add coconut oil to your daily regiment to aid in reducing belly fat, especially after you have completed the *10/14 Fit & Smoothie Cleanse*. You can even cook with coconut oil and put in your smoothies. Cleansing starts on the inside and will eventually heal the body on the outside.

As mentioned, 10/14 Fit & Smoothie Cleanse is uniquely designed to cleanse the entire body from environmental factors, but you must continue detoxing daily by incorporating a routine that works for you after the 10/14. Every organ in the body from the liver to kidney, gallbladder, pancreas, tissues such as the lymph nodes, skin, and feet are detoxed for better health.

Pamper yourself to amplify the cleanse. What good is it to go through a detox and cleanse without pampering yourself? *The 10/14 Fit & Smoothie Cleanse* has a few *"Pampering Detoxing and Cleansing"* recipes that you will love. Do the *"Pampering Detoxing and Cleansing"* 2 to 3 times during the10 days, 4 to 5 times during the 14 days. Body brushing, facial detox, warm bath water detox soak, and foot detox baths are ways to enhance the cleanse. It is amazing how these various detox methods work. *(See Chapters 14 and 15 for additional detoxing and cleanse for the body).* *"Pampering Detoxing and Cleansing"* after the cleanse will be beneficial too.

10/14 Full Cleanse

You should choose to do a full cleanse for 10 days or 14 days. If you choose to do a 10 or 14-day full cleanse, the instructions are the same. Just follow the recipes and don't starve yourself. This is not a DIET! For the next 10 or 14 days, you will have rich creamy smoothies that contain lots of antioxidants with vitamins A, B, C, D, E, and K. Sip on more smoothies during the day if you get hungry, eat recommended snacks, relax, and stay focused. *(Only 3 smoothies a day).* This is needed to keep the body well nourished.

10/14 Moderate Cleanse

The moderate cleanse works the same way as the full cleanse, except you will have two smoothies to replace your meals and have a sensible meal. Follow the recipes and don't starve yourself. This is not a DIET! For the next 10 or 14 days, you will have rich creamy smoothies that contains lots of antioxidants with vitamins A, B, C, D, E, and K. Sip on more smoothies during the day if you get hungry, eat recommended snacks, relax, and stay focus. *(Only 2 smoothies a day).* This is much needed to keep the body well nourished.

Here are four tips for properly drinking smoothies and its effect on the body with protein:

AHY Tip 1: Chew your smoothies for better digestion and to make you feel as if you are eating a meal. It will also make you feel full. I do suggest if you are trying to lose weight, do use the protein, don't use more than the recommended amount. Usually protein is needed to feel full and to build lean muscles, and lose weight. I don't use the protein while doing a full cleanse, but I still feel full. I add more greens. Everyone has a different body make up. If you would like to use the protein add one scoop to the smoothies as recommended.

AHY Tip 2: Taking in protein burns the body fat quicker when you are exercising, but if you do the full-cleanse do less strenuous exercise to heal the body. Relax and allow the body to do just that, heal.

AHY Tip 3: Doing the moderate cleanse prepare detox foods that will help with energy and reduce body fat. If you choose to prepare your own meals, eat baked or broil meats (water fish, chicken) stir fry vegetables in extra virgin olive oil or grapeseed oil and use sodium free seasonings. *(See suggested meal plans).*

AHY Tip 4: If you do brisk walking with the full cleanse, do the protein to burn fat, although adding the protein to the smoothies is optional. For the moderate cleanse, adequate rest and moderate exercise is suggested for your first detox and cleanse.

Hydrating the Body

Drinking water is essential. Drink water for half your body weight daily. Adding more water would be great too! Add squeezed lemon if you don't like plain water. Remember the water formula *(Refer to Chapter 4).* Drink herbal detox teas at least twice a day. Snacks are allowed. Yeah! Eat a snack at mid-morning, afternoon, and at night to cut the hunger pain or sip on smoothie *(See snack list).* I suggest you eat the night snack 2 ½ hours before going to bed. Drink your last smoothie around 8:00 p.m. along with your last bottle of water. This way you wouldn't have probably eliminating urine throughout the night. It also depends on the person's body and their bed time. I usually take in my last detox tea at 9:00 or 10:00 p.m. Drinking water or tea late at night does vary with the person. However, with the release of fluid during the cleanse, my hands or feet didn't swell nor did they feel tight after taking in the right amount fluids every day. Do what works for you! I am sure you will appreciate the benefit of what water does for the body.

Drinking Smoothies, Herbal Teas, Water and Eating Snacks Tips:

AHY Tip 1: ***Don't eat your snacks with your smoothies.*** Wait at least 20 to 25 minutes to eat your snacks or later. If you get hungry, drink more smoothie and drink lots of water.

AHY Tip 2: Eat suggested snacks, but DON'T overdo it! Consume the recommended amount based on the 10/14 plan. Although nuts and seeds are a good source of fat, you don't want to over eat to satisfy your hunger pain. This may hinder your weight loss goal. Remember you are not on a DIET! You are cleansing the body for better health and a jump start to weight loss.

Eliminating Toxins Through Bowel

Eliminating your bowels is important during the cleanse. If you are not able to have a bowel movement on the first full day of the cleanse, you should drink more water, take one or two of the following *Mag 07, Smoothe Move Tea, Super Dieter's Tea, Hyleys Detox Tea, Hyleys Slim Tea Acai Berry and Pomegranate* (Helps Promote Weight Loss) or Salt Water Flush (SWF). Out of these six, you will have the necessary bowel movements that is needed. We are supposed to eliminate waste at least 2-3 times a day. However, after drinking the tea, drink plenty of water.

Tips for Flushing Bowels:

AHY TIP1: If you work in the mornings, skip the SWF. Drink the SWF on a day that you are off work.

AHY Tip 2: If you have high pressure, I suggest **DON'T** do the SWF. Please check with your physician before using this method to eliminate bowel waste.

AHY Tip 3: REMEMBER DRINK WATER! DRINK WATER! Be creative in drinking the water and add fresh lemon or 100% lemon juice.

AHY Tip 4: Drink infused detox water. Infused water can help eliminate toxins and flush body fat.

AHY Tip 5: Consult your physician before starting, changing, or taking any supplements.

Chapter 11

10/14 FIT & SMOOTHIE CLEANSE

Your journey has begun. When I started creating the smoothie recipes for the *10/14 Fit & Smoothie Cleanse*, I had to do a lot of tweaking and revising. It was necessary to test the smoothies several times because I wanted to be sure that the smoothies were creamy, fulfilling and tasty. The smoothies needed to be just right to clean all the organs of the body, especially the liver and the kidneys. When the liver is, fatty and has an overload of toxins, it recirculates through the blood which will cause many dysfunctional problems.

The liver plays a vital role to ensure that the body eliminate heavy toxins that has accumulated over a long period of time. These toxins come from processed foods, chemicals, and environmental toxins. As your liver breaks down hormones like insulin, cortisol, and estrogen, it clears the blood cells when the body is properly cleansed. Therefore, toxins could easily be released through bowel movements and urine.

The kidney's role is to filter out the toxins through the urine so that they can remain healthy. The kidneys can cause a toxic overload with processed foods, excessive chemicals found in beauty and personal care aids, household cleaning products, and environmental factors. The kidneys also produce hormones like the production of red blood cells, blood pressure regulation, calcium metabolism, Vitamin D to strength bones, and enhances immunity. Balancing and regulating the blood pressure and other essential minerals will help the body to restore acid/alkaline balanced with a thorough detox. With these two organs being the most important in detoxification, it is essential that you complete the cleanse to reach your goal for weight loss.

There are 14 delicious recipes for the *10/14 Fit & Smoothie Cleanse*. The purpose of the *10/14 Fit & Smoothie Cleanse* is to detoxify the body for better health and weight loss. You can do the cleanse for 10 days or 14 days. Get it? No matter how you do the days, the weight loss will be evident. The extra 4 days may allow for additional weight loss and total body cleanse. I specifically included on the last 4 days' recipes that will help in healing and cleansing the kidney to regulate the amount of fluids in the body.

Follow the *10/14 Fit & Smoothie Cleanse* to obtain a healthy body and weight loss. Remember for the full cleanse, drink 3 smoothies and for the moderate cleanse drink 2 smoothies per day, drink plenty of water or lemon water, herbal teas, infused water if you desire, and recommended snacks. Add protein if desired to burn fat and to stay full.

Flushing the bowels is essential to avoid constipation. Use one of the recommended products at night after your last smoothie or snack

(Super Dieter's Tea, Mag 07, Hyleys Detox Tea Acai or Pomegranate, or SWF if you do not have high blood pressure) to clear bowels. I only suggest this method only if you are constipated, your bowel has not moved in a day or two, and to clean the intestines. In addition, do not use this method if you work in the mornings, it is not a great experience to be at work and have several bowel movements.

Tips to Get Started On the 10/14 Fit & Smoothie Cleanse:

AHY Tip 1: Take a front and side view picture of yourself before and after the cleanse. Take a head shot photo. Take photos throughout the cleanse and share in the "A Healthier You" group on Facebook, on the website, and Instagram.

AHY Tip 2: Weigh yourself on day 1 and write your daily activities, accomplishments, and feelings in the *"My 10/14 Journey"* in *Chapter 20*.

AHY Tip 3: Don't weigh in the second time until the end of the cleanse. It's important to do this because your weight will fluctuate throughout the cleanse. But if you can't wait to see the progress, go ahead weigh yourself. Keep pushing towards your goal.

AHY Tip: Do the cleanse with a family member or a friend.

AHY Tip 4: Join in with the support group on "A Healthier You" w/Dr. V. Benson on Facebook

https://www.facebook.com/groups/AHealthierYouwDr.V.Benson/

AHY TIP 5: Become "A Healthier You" VIP member on the website.

http://www.ahealthieryou-detoxify-cleansewithdrvbenson.org/

10/14 Fit & Smoothie Cleanse Recipes

Here are the recipes to start your 10/14 Fit & Smoothie Cleanse. Drink and chew your smoothies. If you are doing the full-cleanse take in 3 smoothies a day. For the moderate-cleanse do 2 smoothies a day along with a sensible meal. Drink plenty of water, lemon water, herbal teas and infused water, and eat your recommended snacks.

Day 1 Berry Berry

3 handfuls spinach

1 cup water

1 banana peeled

1 cored green apple (sliced quartered)

1 cup frozen or fresh blueberries

½ cup frozen or Fresh Strawberry

2 tbsps. flaxseeds (Ground or mill)

1 stevia (Optional)

1 scoop protein powder (Optional)

Blend spinach, flaxseeds, and banana with water for 30 secs. Add remainder ingredients and blend for 30 seconds or until smooth.

Day 2 Tropical Green Orange Pineapple

3 handfuls spring mix power greens

½ cup water

½ cup frozen pineapple chunks

1 cup frozen or fresh blueberries

½ orange peeled, deseeded

½ lemon or ½ lime peeled, deseeded

2 tbsps. flaxseeds (Ground or mill)

1 stevia (Optional)

1 scoop protein powder (Optional)

Blend spring mix greens, blueberries, orange, and lemon or lime with water for 60 seconds. Add remain ingredients and blend for 30 seconds or until smooth.

Day 3 Apple Almond

1 handful spinach

2 handfuls spring mix greens

1 ½ cup water

2 cored green apples

1 cup frozen or fresh strawberries

2 tbsps. flaxseeds (Ground or mill)

½ tbsp. lemon juice or ½ lemon squeezed

1 handful plain unsalted almonds

1 stevia (Optional)

1 scoop protein powder (Optional)

Blend spinach, green apple, lemon juice or lemon, and flaxseeds with water for 30 seconds. Add remaining ingredients until smooth.

Day 4 Banana Berry Pineapple

2 handfuls kale

1 handful spinach

1 ½ cup water

1 banana peeled

1 cup frozen mixed berries

½ cup frozen pineapple chunks

1 tbsp. lemon juice or ½ fresh lemon squeezed

2 tbsps. flaxseeds (Ground or mill)

1 stevia (Optional)

1 scoop protein powder (Optional)

Blend spinach, banana, water and flaxseeds until smooth for 30 seconds. Add remainder ingredients and blend for 30 seconds or until smooth. Delicious!!!!!!!

Day 5 Peachy Green Apple

3 handful spring mix power greens

1½ cup water

1 banana peeled

1 cored green apple

2 cups frozen or fresh peaches

1 tbsp. sunflower seeds (Unsalted)

2 tbsps. flaxseeds (Ground or mill)

1 stevia (Optional)

1 scoop protein powder (Optional)

Blend spring mix greens, banana, sunflower seed and flaxseed with water for 30 seconds. Add remainder ingredients and blend for 30 seconds or until smooth.

Day 6 Tropical Pineapple Banana Mango

2 handfuls spinach

1 handful kale

1 ½ cup water

1 cored green apple

2 bananas peeled

1 cup frozen mango

1 ½ cup frozen pineapple chunks

1Tbsp. lemon juice or ½ fresh lemon squeezed

2 tbsps. flaxseeds (Ground or mill)

1 stevia (Optional)

1 scoop protein powder (Optional)

Blend spinach, kale, bananas, and apple, and flaxseeds with water for 30 seconds. Add remainder ingredients and blend for 30 seconds or until smooth.

Day 7 Robust Spicy Green

1 handful spinach

2 handfuls kale

1 ½ cup water

½ cup fresh green seedless grapes

½ small cucumber

1 cored green apple

1 kiwi

1 cup frozen mixed berries

2 celery stalks

3 slices fresh ginger (Washed and skinned) or 1tbsp. ground ginger

1 tbsp. lemon juice or ½ fresh lemon squeezed

2 tbsps. flaxseeds (Ground or mill)

1 scoop protein powder (Optional)

Blend spinach, kale, cucumber, celery stalks, ginger root, flaxseeds with water for 60 seconds. Add to remainder ingredients for 30 seconds or until smooth. GO GREEN!

Day 8 Blueberry Mango Blast

2 handfuls spring mix power greens

1 handful spinach

1 cup water

1 cored green apple

1 cup frozen or fresh blueberries

1 cup frozen mango

1 handful almonds or walnuts

2 tbsps. flaxseeds (Ground or mill)

1 scoop protein powder (Optional)

Blend spring green mix, spinach, cored apple, flaxseeds for 30 seconds. Add the reminder ingredients and blend for 30 seconds or until smooth.

Day 9 Banana Pineapple

3 handfuls spring mix power greens

1 cup of water

1 banana peeled

1 ½ cup frozen pineapple chunks

1 cup fresh red seedless grapes

2 tbsps. flaxseeds (Ground or mill)

1 scoop protein powder (Optional)

Blend spring mix power greens, banana, celery, grapes and flaxseed for 30 seconds. Add other ingredients for additional 30 seconds or until smooth.

Day 10 Berry Mango

1 handful spinach

2 handfuls kale

1 banana peeled

1 ½ cup water

1 cup frozen mixed berries

½ cup frozen mango

2 tbsps. flaxseeds (Ground or mill)

1 stevia (Optional)

1 scoop protein powder (Optional)

Blend spinach, kale, flaxseeds, and banana with water for 30 seconds Add remainder ingredients and blend for 30 seconds or until smooth. Yummy!!

Weighing In

Have you weighed in? If you have reached your goal at day 10, you are now ready to make the "Fat Flush" soup to break the cleanse. Do two smoothies and eat the "Fat Flush" soup for dinner for three days. When you have completed the 3 days for breaking the cleanse, I suggest you use the 5-day detox meals to learn how to eat clean or use the 5-day detox meals as an example to plan your own healthy meals. Drink plenty of water or lemon water, herbal teas, and/or infused water and flush your bowels with the supplements if you become constipated. This will help to maintain the weight loss. If you want to switch to a moderate cleanse still drink 2 smoothies a day and eat a sensible meal. You can restart the 10/14-day full-cleanse in 21 days.

Feel Good About Your Weight Loss?

Got the guts to do more? Challenge yourself! Continue with the 14-day Fit & Smoothie Cleanse. Here are the remainder of 4 days for the *"10/14 Fit & Smoothie Cleanse"*.

Day 11 Apple Carrot Pineapple

3 handfuls spinach

1 cup water

1 cored green apple

1 ½ cup frozen pineapple chunks

½ sliced cucumber

½ orange

½ cup carrots

1 small chopped tomato

3 slices ginger root (Washed and skinned) or 1 tbsp. ground ginger

2 tbsps. flaxseeds (Ground or mill)

1 stevia (Optional)

1 scoop protein powder (Optional)

Blend spinach, carrots, tomato, apple, cucumber, ginger, and flaxseeds with water for 30 seconds. Add remainder ingredients and blend for 30 seconds or until smooth.

Day 12 Green Apple Walnut

3 handfuls spring mix power greens

1 ½ cup water

2 cored green apples

1 cup frozen mixed fruit or (Fresh 5 sliced strawberries, 1 mango chunked, 5 cubed pineapples and 1riped chunked peach) (Deseed mango and peach).

1 handful walnuts (unsalted)

2 tbsps. flaxseeds (Ground or mill)

1 stevia (Optional)

1 scoop protein powder (Optional)

Blend spring mix power greens, green apples, flaxseeds and walnuts for 30 seconds. Add remainder ingredients and blend for 30 seconds or until smooth.

Day 13 Spinach Kale Dark Berry

1 handful spinach

2 handfuls kale

1 cup water

1 banana peeled

1 bunch parsley

1 ½ cup frozen or fresh blueberries

1 cup frozen or fresh blackberries

½ cup red or black grapes

2 tbsps. flaxseeds (Ground or mill)

1 stevia (Optional)

1 scoop protein powder (Optional)

Blend spinach, kale, banana, grapes, and flaxseeds with water for 30 seconds. Add remainder ingredients and blend for 30 seconds or until smooth.

Day 14 Green Apple Cranberries Grapes

3 handfuls spinach

1 cup water

2 cored green apples

1 cup red seedless grapes or green seedless grapes

1½ cup frozen fresh cranberries (pitted cranberries if
fresh)

2 celery stalks

1 handful parsley

1 tsp. cinnamon

1 tsp. turmeric (Ground or root)

1 tbsps. flaxseeds (Ground or mill)

1 stevia (Optional)

1 scoop protein (Optional)

Blend spinach, green apples, grapes, and flaxseeds with water for 30 seconds. Add remainder ingredients and blend for 30 seconds or until smooth.

SNACK RECIPES

Here are the snack recipes. Eat snacks three times a day. Eat the recommended snacks for continuous weight loss.

Apple Peanut Butter or Almond Butter

1 wedged sliced apple

1 tbsp. apple cider vinegar (ACV)

2 tbsps. Peanut butter or almond butter

Directions:

Slice apples and add 1 tbsp. of ACV and toss. Melt the peanut butter or almond butter in the microwave and drizzle over apples.

Tuna Salad

1 cup pack tuna (In water)

1 tbsp. vegan mayonnaise

1 boiled egg (Diced)

½ cored apple (Diced)

Sprinkle with paprika (Optional

This recipe has additional ingredients when you are on the moderate cleanse. *(See Chapter 16).*

Boiled Eggs

Directions:

Two boiled eggs. Cut in halves and add paprika, black pepper, and 1 pinch of sea salt (Optional)

Apple Cucumber Salad

1 diced apple

1 diced cucumber

2 tbsps. Braggs Apple Cider Vinegar (ACV)

2 tbsps. lite raspberry vinaigrette (Optional)

Directions:

Mixed diced apples and cucumber toss in ACV and or lite raspberry vinaigrette.

Cucumber with Cayenne Pepper

1 sliced and peeled cucumber

2 pinches of cayenne pepper

2 tbsps. Bragg's Apple Cider Vinegar (ACV)

Directions:

Toss sliced cucumbers in ACV and sprinkle with pinched cayenne pepper.

Frozen Fruit with ACV

Frozen Mixed Berries

1 cup mixed frozen berries

2 tbsps. Bragg's Apple Cider Vinegar

4 tbsps. water

1 Stevia

1 cup of ice

Makes an icy blended dessert. Refreeze for 10 minutes for harder ice. You can also use fresh lime, lemons frozen blueberries, peaches, strawberries, and pineapples.

Snack list

Raw unsalted nuts: Peanuts, Cashews, Almonds, Walnuts

Eggs

Cucumber

Broccoli

Peanut Butter

Almond Butter

Celery

Tuna

Apples

Carrots

Grapes (handful)

Chapter 12

BREAKING THE CLEANSE

Getting to this step prepares you to continue your journey for eating healthy, losing weight, and maintaining the weight loss. Breaking the cleanse should be simple, but you should control what you eat and when you eat. Over eating can occur because you have not eaten full meals and other food stuff in a while. The "Fat Flush" soup is an ideal meal you can start with breaking the cleanse. The "Fat Flush" is a way to continue your detox and flush more fat from the body as you continue lose weight and gain the best of your health.

It is important that you break your detox-cleanse with ease. The body is still in the healing process. You don't want to introduce foods that you have not eaten in 10-14 days such as fried chicken, French fries, cake, cookies, chips, etc. This will be too harsh on the stomach and it defeats the purpose for cleansing. Your body is now free from toxins and the body is looking forward to the healthy foods that it has acquired within the past 10-14 days.

Start with the "Fat Flush" soup. The soup is a very popular homemade healthy vegetable soup that was created by nutrition experts. You can continue to maintain your healthy lifestyle and lose weight by drinking two smoothies a day, eating a sensible healthy meal, and of course drinking plenty of water along with the herbal detox teas and infused water. You can make your own healthy smoothies, but be careful on adding the fruit. Add less fruit and more green leafy veggies. *(See Chapter 12 for more smoothie recipes).*

Tips for Breaking the Cleanse

AHY Tip 1: Break the cleanse with ease and make it simple by drink 2 smoothies and eating the "Fat Flush" soup.

AHY Tip 2: Starting with the "Fat Flush" soup introduces the body to solid foods that still aids in antioxidants, continuously flushes fat and adds valued nutrients.

AHY Tip 3: Don't over eat whatever you eat and don't struggle in contemplating on what to eat. Your thoughts will signal healthy choices.

AHY Tip 4: Eat slowly and eat small portions for planned meals.

AHY Tip 5: If you have done the 10 or 14-day full cleanse, do a moderate cleanse afterwards. Plan a sensible third meal. You can also do the "Fat Flush" soup for your third meal. Salads and lean meat can be added after breaking the cleanse with the "Fat Flush" soup. You can also add the meat to your soup, like skinless chicken breast or turkey.

AHY Tip 6: Eat healthy snacks if you are continuing your weight loss journey. Keep in mind that your sugar intake should not be more than 5 g per day. Sodium from foods no more than 6 g (2 tsps.).

AHY Tip 7: Eat baked, broiled, grilled, or stir fry lean meats. Stir fry vegetables in extra virgin olive oil, or grapeseed oil. Use seasonings with no sodium or no more than 6 g.

AHY Tip 8: Drink lots of water and add the fresh squeezed lemon or lemon juice in the water. Get plenty of rest and exercise 2-3 times a week. Your body is still healing and processing the new you.

When you have broken your cleanse, start with the "Fat Flush" soup. Drink to two smoothies as a meal replacement and eat the "Fat Flush" soup as the last meal of the day.

Fat Flush Recipe

Ingredients:

1 medium sweet potato, peeled and cut into 1" cubes

3 carrots, peeled and sliced

1 stalk celery, diced

1 small yellow onion, diced

1 clove garlic, minced

Pinch of Kosher or sea salt, to taste

1/2 teaspoon black pepper

1/8 teaspoon allspice

1 teaspoon paprika

1 bay leaf

2 (15 ounce) cans kidney beans, drained and rinsed (optional, black or navy beans)

4 cups vegetable broth, low-sodium

1 (14.5 oz.) can diced tomatoes (no salt added), *this is an optional ingredient

4 cups baby spinach, loosely packed

1 tablespoon plus 1 teaspoon extra-virgin olive oil, optional, for serving (1/2 teaspoon per serving)

Directions:

Add all ingredients, except spinach and olive oil, to the slow cooker. Cover and cook on low 6 to 8 hours, or until the vegetables are tender. Add spinach, stir and continue cooking just until wilted, approximately 5 minutes. Serve and enjoy!

Tip: Try a thicker soup, after 5 hours of cooking, by removing 1 cup of soup, along with ingredients, mash ingredients with a fork, return to the slow cooker, stir and continue cooking 1 to 3 hours. When serving, drizzle a little (optional) olive oil over each bowl of soup.

Note: Olive oil helps the body absorb nutrients more efficiently and supports a healthy digestive system. Add meat if you desire (Skinless chicken breast or turkey is an option).

This "Fat Flush" soup recipe was inspired by JJ. Smith "10 Green Smooth Cleanse".

Chapter 13

AFTER THE CLEANSE: 5-DAY DETOX MEALS

Although you will continue to detox and cleanse the body daily to stay on the right track for your weight loss goal, or to maintain, you must continue to eat nutritional detoxed meals on a moderate cleanse. I have provided for you a *5-Day Detox Meal Plan* to get you started with healthy eating after the full-cleanse. However, you can choose to do one of the three things to maintain the weight loss until the next full cleanse:

1. Prepare the 5-day detox meals for 5 days.
2. Eat the "Fat Flush" soup for three days and replace 2 meals with smoothies. Drink the lemon water and or do the ACV Cran-Pomegranate cocktail to flush belly fat.
3. Do a moderate cleanse. Drink 2 smoothies to replace two meals and make your own sensible dinner.

Always add flaxseeds or chia seeds to your smoothies. Flaxseeds provides Omega 3 fatty acids the "good fat" antioxidant, fiber, and heart healthy. Chia seeds also contains Omega 3, fiber, protein, adds fullness and thickening to the smoothie. If you want to continue to lose weight, drink 1-2 smoothies a day and follow the exact recipes for detox meals. Some people like making their own meals. If you decide to prepare your own meals during the moderate cleanse, eat light meals that are low in sodium, use good fat oils (*Extra Virgin Olive Oil, Coconut Oil, Grapeseed Oil*) green leafy veggies, baked, broiled, or grilled fish *(Fresh Water)* turkey, chicken or healthy detox soups and salads. See table for other suggested foods to prepare your light meals. I have included more delicious smoothies found in *Chapter 20*. You can create your own smoothies (using the right proportions of fruit and vegetables) or use some of the smoothies from the 10/14 Fit & Smoothie Cleanse.

MORE FLUSHING AFTER THE CLEANSE

During the moderate cleanse, you may have to empty your urine several times during the day and night. Know that you are flushing the kidneys, liver, and body fat. Flushing the liver is the key to losing weight. Adding more water to flush the "fat away". Also, water provides more energy because it contains oxygen. When your body flushes the fluid often, it is a sign that your body is getting rid of toxins through urine, bowel, and even sweat. You must continue drinking the recommended water amount per body weight, the Mag 07, or Dieter's Tea, or SWF to eliminate your bowels, especially if you have not released the bowel within 24 hours. It's good to go 2-3 times a day. Remember this is not a DIET! You are now learning how to eat the right foods at this point.

EVERY DAY DETOX

Continue to detox and cleanse the body daily with good clean foods, flushing with water, herbal detox teas, and infused water. I discovered that detoxing every day has led to more weight loss as well as maintaining my weight. However, it helps to continue the weight loss before doing another round of full cleanse.

Stretching and twisting the upper body torso in the morning and evenings will help relieve stress and toxins. Body brushing, detoxing the skin and feet also helps in releasing more toxins. You can do this 2-3 times a week. Your body will appreciate the outcome when more toxins is released this way.

Tips for Everyday Detox:

AHY Tip 1: Drink lots of water to move toxins and to have regular bowel movements.

AHY Tip 2: Drink herbal detox teas, ACV and Cran- Pomegranate cocktail, and infused water.

AHY Tip 3: Enjoy a meal replacement with a smoothie of choice. Leafier greens and less fruit.

AHY Tip 4: Plan your meals carefully.

AHY Tip 5: Eat and chew your food slowly for better digestion.

AHY Tip 6: Elimination is still important 2-3 times a day. Take Mag O7, Smoothe Move Tea, Super Dieter's Tea, Hyleys Detox Tea, Hyleys Slim Tea Acai Berry and Pomegranate (Helps promote weight loss and removes bowel).

AHY Tip 7: Avoid process foods and eat cleaner foods. Eat healthy snacks. Check the labels before buying. Look for sugar and salt content. 5 grams of sugar and 6 grams of salt per day.

AHY Tip 8: Eating clean eliminates toxins. Buy organic fruits and vegetables. Fresh fruits and vegetables must be thoroughly washed repeatedly before eating. (Always wash organic/fresh fruits and vegetables).

AHY Tip 9: Avoid alcohol. Alcohol is toxic to the body. If you drink any alcohol do one day of full cleanse to get rid of the toxins.

AHY Tip 10: Exercise, detox soak baths, and foot detox weekly to amplify the cleanse.

AHY Tip 11: Keep the digestive tract healthy with probiotics and coconut oil.

AHY Tip 12: Pray and meditate morning and evening, do deep breathing exercising, and morning stretches.

AHY Tip 13: If you gain weight while detoxing every day or you plateau, refer to the *10/14 Fit & Smoothie Cleanse* plan to get you started again. Drink more water and exercise.

AHY Tip 14: Get plenty of rest.

It takes time to get it right, but you will reach your goal.

EVERY DAY DETOXING FOODS

Fruit	Leafy Greens & Vegetables	Seeds & Nuts Boost (unsalted)	Oils	Spices	Drinks
Apples	Kale	Almonds	Olive	Cayenne	Apple Cider
Bananas	Spinach	Sesame Seeds	Coconut	Cinnamon	Vinegar
Blackberries	Arugula	Walnuts	Grapeseed	Turmeric	Cranberry
Blueberries	Collards	Peanuts		Ginger	Pomegranate
Cantaloupes	Spring Greens	Cashew		Basil	
Grapefruit	Artichokes	Flaxseed			Herbal Teas
Honey Dew	Beets	Chia Seed			Peppermint
Melon	Celery	Hemp Seed			Chamomile
Mango	Asparagus	Sunflower Seeds			Skin Tea (Yogi
Strawberries	Onions				Cinnamon vanilla
Raspberries	Fennel				or Skin Detox)
Pears	Garlic				Plant Based Foods
Grapes	Cilantro				Boost
Kiwi	Parsley				Protein Powder
Nectarines	Watercress				Seaweed
Oranges	Cauliflower				Wheat Grass
Papayas	Broccoli				Lemon Grass
Peaches	Cabbage				
Pineapples	Swiss Chard				
Goji Berries					
Cranberries					
Pomegranate					
Avocados					
Lime					
Lemons					
Watermelons					

See *Chapter 20* to learn how to build your own healthy detox smoothies to maintain efficient weight loss and your optimal health. Have your family and friends to join in with you. This could be the best lifestyle change you have ever endured.

EAT LEAN MEATS: AFTER THE CLEANSE

Meats contain proteins and takes longer to digest. The body needs protein to produce metabolism. Without lean meats, it slows the metabolism and changes your moods. Eating lean meats build muscle protein and continued weight loss. Lean meats contain B-vitamin complex, zinc, and Omega 3 and should be eaten with a balanced diet. Cook your meats by baking, broiling, grilling, or stir fry. You also add your meats to homemade soups and with side vegetables such as broccoli, asparagus, collard greens, green beans, kale greens, spinach, and other green leafy vegetables. Add quinoa rice or baked sweet potato. Even a green salad with tomatoes, green or red onions, cucumbers, and light vinaigrette is a delicious meal. **Lean meats:** *Chicken (skinless), turkey, fish (fresh water), top loin, sirloin tips, ground round or loin beef, pork and lamb loin, and tuna.*

Eating lean meat tips:

AHY Tip 1: After you have successfully reached your goal eat lean meats to add in the protein.

AHY Tip 2: Eat chicken, turkey, fish (fresh water) or tuna for the moderate cleanse. Tuna can be eating on the full-cleanse as a snack too.

Chapter 14

DETOX YOUR FEET SOAK

Remember when I said the *"10/14 Fit & Smoothie Cleanse"* will include *"Pamper Detoxing and Cleansing"*? Detoxing and cleansing your skin is an excellent way to eliminate toxins. Although there are several other ways to detox your feet, here are a few recipes to detox those tired aching feet, eliminate toxins, remove the dead skin cells, and roughness. Sweat out your toxins by adding ginger root to the mix. This makes soft supple foot skin. Enjoy the pampering with a cup of hot herbal detox tea.

Detox Your Feet Recipes!

Recipe 1
Warm to Hot Water Bath
1/3 Cup Epsom Salt
1/3 Cup Sea Salt
1 Cup Apple Cider Vinegar (ACV)
1/4 Cup Baking Soda
3 Tbsp. Grounded Ginger Root

Directions:

Remove toe nail polish. Mix all dry ingredients in a bowl. Pour in your ACV in slowly to the dry ingredients and mix. In the running water pour your mixture. Soak your feet for 15-25minutes.

(Optional): Use a pedicure tool set after 10 minutes of soaking remove dead skin cells from the cuticle of the toes, heel, and sole of the feet *(use the correct tool in the pedicure tool set)*. Place your feet back in the solution for 10-15 minutes more. Rinse with warm water and pat dry. Moisturize with coconut oil, Shea butter, petroleum jelly or Vaseline.

===

Recipe 2

1/4 cup Sea Salt or Himalayan Salt
1/4 cup Epsom Salt
1/4 cup Baking Soda
1/3 cup Apple Cider Vinegar (ACV)
Favorite essential oils if desired (I use 10 drops of peppermint or lavender)

Directions:

Remove toe nail polish. Dissolve Salt, Epsom salt, and baking soda in boiling water in a quart size jar and set aside. Fill tub with warm/hot water and add apple cider vinegar. Pour salt mixture in and add essential oils if using (*http://wellnessmama.com/8331/detox-bath-recipes/*). Soak feet for 15-25 minutes or until desired.

(Optional): Use a pedicure tool set after 10 minutes of soaking remove dead skin cells from the cuticle of the toes, heel, and sole of the feet *(use the correct tool in the pedicure tool set).* Place your feet back in the solution for 10-15 minutes more. Rinse with warm water and pat dry. Moisturize with coconut oil, Shea butter, petroleum jelly or Vaseline.

===

Recipe 3

Warm or Hot Water

¼ Cup Coarse Sea Salt

1 Cup of Lemon Juice or Orange Juice (Optional: Fresh Squeezed Lemon or Orange)

½ Cup Apple Cider Vinegar (ACV)

2 Tsp Ground Ginger

Directions:

Remove toe nail polish. Mix all dry ingredients in a bowl. Pour in your ACV and lemon juice or orange juice slowly to the dry ingredients and mix. In the running water pour your mixture. Soak your feet for 25 – 30 minutes or until desired.

(Optional): Use a pedicure tool set after 10 minutes of soaking remove dead skin cells from the cuticle of the toes, heel, and sole of the feet *(use the correct tool in the pedicure tool set).* Place your feet back in the solution for 10-15 minutes more. Rinse with warm water and pat dry. Moisturize with coconut oil, Shea butter, petroleum jelly or Vaseline.

Chapter 15

DETOX YOUR SKIN

The skin is the largest organ of the body. If the opening of the skin is exposed to any toxins or impurities from the environment, the body will easily become toxic on the inside and outside. Skin is the first line of defense and protects us from environmental factors, including bacteria and viruses. However, the skin can still absorb toxins because of open pores and open cavities of the body such the nasal and oral cavity.

Toxins can find a way to enter the body and eventually manifest itself in our blood stream. Then our cells become damage and therefore we suffer with various skin disorders and diseases. Cleansing and detoxing your skin is so important. We must protect our skin from the overbearing of heat and cold. Exposure to insulation, formaldehyde, aerosols, and household cleaning chemicals will also cause many problems internally and externally that will eventually build up toxins in the body. Excessive sun exposure causes the changes that we believe is a normal part of aging and we protect ourselves with a sunscreen, or makeup with sunscreen, and a moisturizer to avoid these problems.

Over exposure of ultraviolet rays from the sun can be very damaging to the skin that can cause pre-cancerous and cancer cells, fine and coarse wrinkles, elastosis *(damaged elastic and collagen causing sagging and wrinkles)*, sallowness *(yellow discoloration of the skin)*, benign tumors freckles, blemishes, skin lesions *(acne, pimples, fissures)*, and age spots. Antioxidants found in fruits, vegetables, and coconut oil protects us from sun damage which may have some effect to keep our skin from aging or being damage even further. Cold combined with low humidity causes dry skin, dandruff, and irritability that can also damage the skin. Here to again, eliminating toxins from the body with a weekly detox can restore the skin to its normal state.

Releasing toxins from the largest organ will eliminate free radicals that causes skin disorders and diseases such as acne, eczema, psoriasis, itchy, dry, scaly, and oily skin, pores, blackheads, pimples, white heads, razor bumps, scabies, fungus, and cellulitis. With daily detoxing the entire body, you will see a difference in your skin when you start eliminating refined sugars, white bread, white pasta, processed foods, caffeinated drinks such as soda, coffee, and oils such as vegetable, canola, soy, and cotton.

If you are having constant bloating, back pain, allergies, trouble relaxing, constipation, itchy skin, and have ever had a fever, a "Detox Bath Soak" is in order. A "Detox Bath Soak" is to eliminate toxins from the body even more. Along with prayer and meditation, healthy eating, drink water smoothies, herbal detox teas, lemon water, apple cider vinegar cocktails, and body brushing, I am sure you will be on your way to a good bill of health.

Detoxing the Skin Tips:

AHY Tip 1: Detox the skin 2-3 times a week to have supple smooth and rejuvenating skin.

AHY Tip 2: Eliminate excessive sun and heat exposure.

AHY TIP 3: If you are in the sun for long periods of time use a sunscreen, but remember to detox the skin by simply using the detox skin recipes.

AHY Tip 4: Detox and cleanse your skin 2-3 times a week with using the "Detox Bath Soak" recipe.

AHY Tip 5: Drink warm or hot lemon water daily to flush the liver which will help to remove toxins.

AHY Tip 6: Do facial lemon water wash and use a non-abrasive skin cleanser for your skin type.

AHY Tip7: After a full cleanse continue to drink lots of water. Drink smoothies 1-2 times a day, and 1000 mg of coconut oil. When you are detoxing the body, your skin will start to glow. Your skin will clear up from infections and inflammations that you may have while eliminating toxins. But you must be consistent.

==

Detox Bath Soak Recipe

1/3 Cup Epsom Salt

½ Cup Coarse Sea Salt

2 Tsp. Ground Ginger

1 Tbsp. Fresh Lemon Juice

Directions:

Combine all ingredients in a bowl. Draw a warm bath water and pour the mixture in the tub. The running water will help mix the ingredients. Soak 20-30 minutes.

Suskind, R. R., (2009). "Environment and the skin". Environmental Health Perspectives. Vol. 20, pp. 27-37. 1977. Retrieved from http://www.pubmedcentral.nih.gov/picrender.fcgi?artid=1637330 &blobtype=pdf

Pilang, M., (Video file). Which sunscreen is better: Spray or lotion? Retrieved from http://www.webmd.com/beauty/sun-exposure-skin-cancer#

Chapter 16

TRANSITIONING INTO A MODIFIED CLEANSE

5 Day Detox Dinners and Desserts

Are you ready to introduce more clean food to your body? Use the 5-Day Detox Dinners and Desserts plan after the 10/14 Fit & Smoothie Cleanse. These recipes can be used as a moderate cleanse. Drink 2 smoothies a day of your choice for breakfast and lunch, healthy snacks plus a sensible dinner, and desserts *(See Chapter 20 for more smoothies or choose the smoothies from the 10/14 or you can do your own)*. Be careful on adding more fruit than leafy greens. I have prepared for you 5 days of detox dinners and desserts just to get you started.

You don't want to revert to your old eating habits. I made these recipes many times to continue my weight loss and to maintain clean healthy eating. You want to stay hydrated. Drink plenty of water and lemon water. Drink infused water to add flavor, ACV cocktails (always drink 16 oz. ACV cocktail twice a day) and detox teas to continue to maintain or lose weight until your next full cleanse.

Day 1

Green Apple Walnut Salad

1 handful spring mixed power greens and ½ cup baby spinach

1 boiled egg sliced over salad

1 cored sliced green apple

6 sliced strawberries

1 handful walnuts or pecans

Salad Dressing

¼ cup olive oil

¼ cup Braggs apple cider vinegar

½ lemon or 4 tbsps. lemon juice

¼ tsp. sea salt

1 tsp. garlic powder

1 tsp. onion powder

1 tsp. Cajun spice

1 tsp. Cajun spice (McCormick Perfect Pinch)

1 tsp salad supreme (McCormick Perfect Pinch)

Directions:

Blend all ingredients in a bowl and pour over salad.

Dessert: See snack list for dinner

Drink: 1 cup Detox Tea and Infused Water (See infused water Chapter 17)

Day 2

Bake Chicken w/ Brown Rice

2-4oz baked chicken breast

1 tsp. parsley flakes

3 tbsps. olive, coconut or grapeseed oil

1 tsp. garlic powder

1 Tsp. Onion Powder

¼ tsp. black pepper

1 tsp. dried basil leaves

1 cup string beans (No salt)

1 cup water

½ cup brown rice

Directions:

Baked Chicken Prep: Coat chicken with 1 tbsp. olive, coconut or grade seed oil. Use a Ziploc bag to mix seasonings and rub on the chicken breast. Place chicken on parchment paper fold down the ends of the parchment paper like a bag to enclose the chicken. Bake for 25-30 minutes or until golden brown.

String Bean Prep: On low heat pour 2 tbsps. olive, coconut, or grape seed oil into a small boiler. Add garlic and onion powder, string beans and stir for 5 minutes. Add water and boil for 10 minutes. Boil brown rice until cooked and strain off water. Place baked chicken over the bed of brown rice.

Dessert: (Make the following dessert or see snack list and choose snack)

Creamy Pineapple Delight

1 cup almond or coconut milk (Unsweetened)

1 cup frozen pineapple

1tsp. vanilla extract (without alcohol content)

2 packets Stevia

Blend ingredients in a blender until creamy like ice cream.

Drink*:* 1 cup detox tea and/or infused water

Day 3

Sautéed Spinach w/Roma Tomato

2 cups spinach

¼ tsp. sea salt

1 tsp. garlic powder

1 tsp. onion powder

1 tbsp. olive or grapeseed Oil

½ tsp. flake parsley or ¼ chopped fresh parsley

1 sliced Roma tomato

2 boiled eggs sliced

Sautéed spinach in olive oil or grape seed oil. Add seasonings and heat for 10-15 minutes. Sautéed Roma tomato the same as the spinach and add parsley.

Apple Cucumber Salad

½ diced cucumber

1 cored green apple

Light raspberry vinaigrette (Watch the nutrition value for the dressing. Should contain 5g or less of sugar)

Directions:

Toss diced cucumber and green apple in light raspberry vinaigrette.

Dessert: See snack list and/or have 1 cup detox tea or infused water.

Day 4

Baked Fish or Tuna Salad

2-4oz baked fish (Tilapia)

1 cup broccoli

1 tsp. olive, coconut or grapeseed oil

1 cup carrots

Pinch Sea Salt

½ tsp. garlic powder

½ tsp. onion powder

¼ tsp. paprika

¼ tsp. black pepper

Directions:

Baked Fish: Prep: Add a light coat to the fish with olive oil, coconut or grape seed oil. Use a Ziploc bag to mix garlic and powder and rub on the fish. Place fish in parchment paper fold down the parchment like a bag to enclose the fish. Cook for 15 minutes.

Steamed Vegetables: Steam and season broccoli in sea salt and garlic powder. Steam and no season needed for carrots. Cook vegetables 10 minutes.

Tuna Salad

1 cup pack tuna (In water)

1 tbsp. vegan mayonnaise

1 boiled egg (Diced)

½ cored apple (Diced)

10 seedless grapes (Sliced in halves)

1 tsp. chopped pecans (Optional)

1 tsp. sweet relish

1 stevia (optional)

Stir the vegan mayonnaise into the tuna Add diced eggs and pickle relish. Stir in the cored apple, grapes, pecans, and Stevia. Sprinkle paprika to garnishment.

Apple Kiwi Salad

1 cup spinach or mixed green

1 cored green apple

1 sliced kiwi

¼ cup raisins (Optional)

Salad Dressing

¼ cup olive oil

¼ cup Braggs vinegar

½ lemon or 4 tbsp. lemon juice

¼ tsp. sea salt

1 tsp. garlic powder

1 tsp. onion Powder

1 tsp. Cajun spice (McCormick Perfect Pinch)

1 tsp. salad supreme (McCormick Perfect Pinch)

OPTIONAL: Light Raspberry Vinaigrette can be used for salad.

Blend in a bowl and pour over salad.

Dessert: 1 Cup grapes or 1 bag of Skinny popcorn

Drink: 1 Cup Detox Tea and Infused Water)

Day 5

Grilled Chicken with Stir Fry Kale Greens

2-4 oz. grilled chicken

2 cups kale

½ red pepper

¼ cup cut scallions

1 tbsp. olive or coconut or grapeseed oil (Grilled chicken and kale)

½ tsp. sea salt (Grilled chicken and kale)

¼ tsp. black pepper (Grilled chicken)

1 tsp. garlic powder (Grilled chicken and kale)

1 tsp. minced garlic

1 tsp. onion powder (Grilled chicken and kale)

Directions:

Grilled Chicken Prep: Coat grill chicken with olive oil, coconut or grape seed oil and add seasoning. Grill for 15-20 minutes or until no redness is shown. Stir fry kale in olive, coconut, grapeseed oil. Add dice red peppers and scallions. Add seasoning and cook for 10-15 minutes.

Green Salad

2 cups spring mixed power greens

1 diced Roma tomato

½ cup raw carrots (Chopped or diced)

¼ raisins or ½ cup grapes

¼ cup sesame seeds

Salad Dressing

¼ cup olive oil

¼ cup Braggs vinegar

½ lemon or 4 tbsp. lemon juice

¼ tsp. sea salt

1 tsp. garlic powder

1 tsp. onion powder

1 tsp. Cajun spice (McCormick Perfect Pinch)

1 tsp. salad supreme (McCormick Perfect Pinch)

OPTIONAL: Light Raspberry Vinaigrette can be used for salad

Dessert:

Walnut Cinnamon Apple Bake

1/8 tsp. cinnamon

1/8 tsp. nutmeg

1/8 vanilla extract (Without the alcohol content)

1 tbsp. lemon juice

1 green apple sliced

½ handful walnuts or pecans

Add Stevia to taste

Directions:

Toss all ingredients in a bowl and baked at 350 for 15-20 minutes.

Drink: 1 cup detox tea and infused water

Chapter 17

DETOX HERBAL TEAS & INFUSED WATER RECIPES

Detox Herbal Teas

Drink the apple cider vinegar tea before drinking your smoothies and eating meals on a moderate cleanse. Drink 2-3 times a day. You can drink warm or cold or drink as a hot tea.

Apple Cider Vinegar Cocktail Tea

4 tbsp. Bragg apple cider vinegar (ACV) (With the mother. The brown residue at the bottle.)

1 bottle of water (500 mL)

1 lemon or 4 tbsp. lemon juice

1 pinch of cayenne pepper for fat burning and more energy

1 Stevia

Directions:

Add all ingredients in a glass, stir and add stevia.

Apple Cider Vinegar Berry Cocktail Tea

4 tbsp. Braggs apple cider vinegar (ACV) (With the mother. The brown residue at the bottom of the bottle.)

1 cup frozen mixed berries

1 bottle of water (500 mL)

1 lemon peeled or 4 tbsp. lemon juice

1 Stevia

Directions:

Blend all ingredients in a blender.

Ginger Tea I

1 cup Water

2 slices ginger root (Washed, skin and grated) or 1 tbsp. ginger grounded

½ lemon squeezed

1 Stevia

You can prep this tea in two ways:

Prep I: Wash the skin of the ginger root, skin and add to hot boiled water. Steep the ginger in the hot water for 2-3 minutes. Discard the ginger root. Add Stevia.

Prep II: If you are using ground ginger add 1tbsp. Pour the ginger mixture in a cup and add hot water. Add the tea bag and steep the tea by covering the cup for 2 minutes. Add stevia for sweetness. Drink and feel the warmth and sensation of the smooth tea as you drink.

Ginger Tea II

1 bag detox tea (For a stronger tea add an addition bag)

2 slices ginger root or 1 tbsp. ground ginger)

½ lemon squeezed

Directions:

Prep I: Wash and peel ginger root place in blender to liquefy. Strain the ginger to obtain the liquid portion. Discard the left-over residue of the ginger. Add ginger and tea bag to hot water. Steep the ginger in the hot water for 2-3 minutes. Add Stevia.

Prep II: If you are using ground ginger add 1tbsp. Pour the ginger mixture in a cup and add hot water. Add tea bag steep the tea by covering the cup for 2 minutes. Add stevia for sweetness. Drink and feel the warmth and sensation of the smooth tea as you drink.

.

Orange Lemon Tea

1 cup water

1 orange

½ lemon squeezed or ¼ cup lemon juice

1 tsp. cinnamon

1 Stevia

Directions:

Remove seeds from the orange and lemon and squeeze into a cup of water. Add cinnamon and heat for 3 minutes. Let it steep and add stevia. Add another stevia for desired taste.

Blueberry Tea

1-2 cups water

1 cup frozen blueberries

½ lemon squeezed or ¼ Cup lemon juice

1 Stevia

Directions:

Puree frozen blueberries in blender with water. Pour blueberries into a cup of water with squeezed lemon and heat for 3 minutes or drink cold after blending. If drinking hot let it steep for 2 minutes. If drinking cold leave in the refrigerator for 25 minutes. Add ice if drinking cold. Add stevia for desired taste.

Green Turmeric Tea

1 ¼ cup water

1 bag green Tea (Decaffeinated)

½ lemon squeezed or 1 tbsp. lemon juice

1tsp turmeric (Ground)

1-2 slices ginger root (Wash and peeled. Place in blender or 1 tbsp.

ground ginger)

1 Stevia

Prep: Use one ¼ cup of water and grind in a blender. Strain grinded ginger and discard the residue. Add the liquid portion of ginger or ground ginger to the 1 cup of water. Heat the water with ginger. Add the tea bag to heated water and steep for 2-3 minutes. Stir in turmeric and lemon or lemon juice and heat as desired. Add stevia for sweetness. Drink and feel the warmth and sensation of the smooth tea as you drink.

Cranberry Orange Tea

1 cup water

1 cup cranberries

½ orange deseeded

1 tsp. cinnamon

1 Stevia

Directions:

Blend cranberries and water in blender. Removed seeds and squeezed the orange in mixture. Add cinnamon and stevia. Heat for three minutes and steep for 1 ½ minutes. For cold tea place in the refrigerator for 25 minutes or overnight.

Cinnamon Mint Tea

1 cup water

5 mint leaves

1 tsp. cinnamon

1 Stevia

Directions:

Heat water and add mint leaves. Remove leaves after 3 minutes. Add cinnamon to hot water. Cover and steep for 2-3 minutes.

Infused Water Recipes

Drink infused water to hydrate the body. Blending various flavors can help with flushing body fat, boost energy, and decrease belly fat. Enjoy these recipes to add to your daily weight loss goals and weight maintenance. Refrigerate 12 to 24 hours to get the full enhanced flavor of the infused water.

Lemon Mint

1 quart water

1 sliced lemon

10 mint leaves

½ sliced cucumber

Strawberry Orange

1 quart water

1 sliced orange peeled

10 halved sliced strawberries

Blueberry Hill

1 quart water

½ cup blueberries

10 halved sliced strawberries

Lemon Lime

1 quart water

1 sliced orange peeled

½ sliced lemon peeled

½ sliced lime peeled

Lemon Raspberry

1 quart water

½ cup raspberry

½ sliced lemon peeled

4 mint leaves

Apple Pineapple

1 quart water

12 slices pineapple chunks

½ sliced orange peeled

10 slices cantaloupe

Ginger Orange Pineapple

1 quart water

1 tbsp. ground ginger

½ sliced orange peeled

½ cup pineapple chunks

Basil Lemon Strawberry

1 quart water

½ sliced lemon peeled

½ cup strawberries

¼ tsp. fresh or ground basil

Watermelon Pineapple

1 quart water

1 cup watermelon cubed

½ cup pineapple chunks

½ sliced lemon peeled

¼ cup raspberry

Strawberry Orange Raspberry

1 quart water

½ cup sliced strawberries

½ cup raspberry

½ orange slices

Cinnamon Orange Mint

1 quart water

1 tsp. cinnamon

½ sliced orange peeled

6 mint leaves

Pineapple Blueberry

1 quart water

1 cup pineapple chunks

½ blueberries

½ sliced lemon peeled

Raspberry Pineapple

1 quart water

½ cup raspberry

½ pineapple chunks

Blueberry Green Apple

1 quart water

½ cup blueberry

1 sliced green apple

Pineapple Mint Orange

1 quart water

½ cup pineapple chunks

10 mint leaves

½ sliced orange

Turmeric Tangerine

1 quart water

1 sliced tangerine

1tsp. ground ginger

Mango Blackberry Lime

1 quart water

½ cup mango

½ sliced lime peeled

½ cup blackberries

Cherry Ginger Mint

1 quart water

½ cup dark red cherries

10 mint leaves

1tsp. ground ginger

Blackberry Blueberry Mint

1 quart water

½ cup blackberries

½ cup blueberries

5 mint leaves

Apple Orange

1 quart water

1 sliced apple

½ sliced orange peeled

5 cinnamon sticks

Cinnamon Pear Ginger

1 quart water

1 sliced pear

1 tsp. fresh grated ginger

5 cinnamon sticks

Mango Strawberry

1 quart water

½ cup mango

½ cup strawberries

½ cucumber sliced

Spicy Lemon Lime Mint

1 quart water

½ lemon sliced peeled

½ lime sliced peeled

5 mint leaves

2 tsps. fresh ginger

Orange Red Grapes

1 quart water

1 sliced orange peeled

½ cup sliced red grapes

Watermelon Cherry Strawberry

1 quart water

½ cup watermelon cubes

½ cup sliced cherries

½ sliced strawberries

Chapter 18

A HEALTHIER YOU SIX TIER PLAN

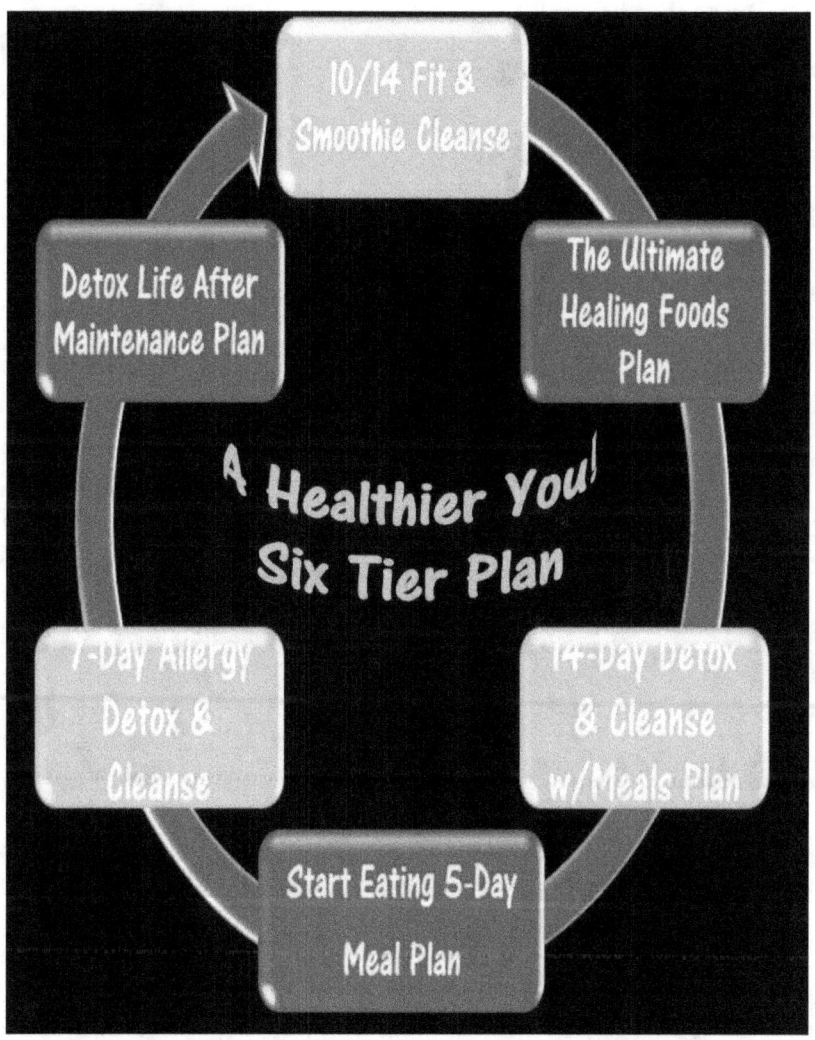

About the Six Tier Plans

A Healthier You Six Tier Plans will help your body in every area for optimal health. Here is an overview of the different plans.

10/14 Fit & Smoothie Cleanse – A detox and cleanse plan for weight loss. You can do this plan for 10 days or 14 days. The *10/14 Fit & Smoothie* is designed to help you with weight loss. As you detoxing and cleanse you will be able to decrease fatigue, memory loss, bloating, swelling, and PMS. This plan can also aid in decreasing high blood pressure, hypertension, and high cholesterol, which increases as weight is gained with unhealthy eating. You will be able to eliminate stress, sugar, and carb cravings that causes us to gain weight. You can lose-up 15 or more pounds following this plan. *(Weight loss will vary with the person)*. The maintenance plan will help with continued weight loss after the *10/14 Fit & Smoothie Cleanse*.

The Ultimate Healing Foods Plan – Change your eating habits for a life time with this plan. The goal for this plan is to decrease body inflammation due to over worked worn out cells that are trying to repair themselves. The *"Ultimate Healing Foods"* plan is designed for you and your family to start eating the right foods to avoid unwanted chronic illness like diabetes, autism, osteoporosis, prevent cancer, hypertension, fibromyalgia, high cholesterol, fibroids, arthritis, impotence, Alzheimer's, digestive disorders, and more. The Ultimate Healing Foods Plan can even work to revert chronic illnesses just by eating the right foods. The plan also benefits in avoiding excessive weight gain, fatigue, headaches, infections, memory loss or fog, PMS, bloating, edema and much more trouble signs of a toxic body. *(The plan includes "Detox Life After Maintenance Plan.")*

14-Day Detox and Cleanse w/Meals – A detox and cleanse plan that works in two parts for weight loss. The first 7 days of the plan is a full-cleanse that include smoothies, herbal teas, and snacks, 5 days of moderate cleanse with prepared home meals of nutritious recipes, followed by 2 - days on a full-cleanse. This plan aids in weight loss, decreasing high blood pressure, hypertension, and high cholesterol from which is increased with weight gain and unhealthy eating. You will be able to eliminate stress, fatigue, memory loss or fog, sugar and carb cravings that causes us to gain weight. You can lose-up to 15 or more pounds following this plan. *(Weight loss varies with the person).*

Start Eating 5-Day Meal Plan – A 5-Day Meal Plan will help you to start eating right and lose weight. The plan will also help you to continue detoxing and cleansing your body. This plan can be used in conjunction with the 14 Day Detox and Cleanse plan. The plan includes meals, herbal teas, infused water recipes, snacks, and desserts.

7-Day Allergy Plan – The 7-Day Allergy Detox and Cleanse is a great way to remove toxins from the body that causes airborne allergies. The detox and cleanse can be used to decrease bacteria and viruses that causes inflammation and upper respiratory infections due to hay fever, postnasal drip, sinus infection, sinus headaches, sore throat, strep throat, and ear infections.

Detox After Life Maintenance Plan – The most robust plan ever! A great plan where you can choose what you want to eat to maintain your optimal health. The plan focuses on healthy meals, desserts, and snack recipes for the whole family. It is a guided plan that help you to select restaurant food choices, make your own herbal teas, and infused waters. Learn how to stay clean and lean with the assistance of personal coaching. The plan also offers exclusive benefits for being a VIP Member with "A Healthier You!

Other Healthy Food Plans

21-Day Daniel Fast Plan – *"I ate no pleasant food, no meat or wine came into my mouth, nor did I anoint myself at all, till three whole weeks were fulfilled"* (Daniel 10:2-3). If you do the Daniel Fast with your church family at the beginning of each new year, this is a great plan for you. Lots' of mouthwatering recipes to get you through 21 days as you pray and meditate to ask God for a deeper understanding and changes for your life. Although you are not focusing on weight loss during this time, it does aid in losing a few pounds. This plan helps you to prepare delicious meals for breakfast, lunch, and dinner including desserts and snacks that are very healthy for you and the entire family to enjoy.

3-Day Turbo Intensity "Jump Start to Weight Loss"- This 3-day jump start to weight loss plan is very intense. It is designed to help you lose up to 5 pounds or more in 3 days. The plan includes the "Fat Flush" soup recipe. The "Fat Flush" soup is an all-vegetable soup loaded with antioxidants to help flush fat.

Healthier Kids Eating Plan - Kids like smoothies too! The plan is to introduce kids to healthy eating and snacking through their growing years. Kids can also make fun snacks with a little help from their parents. What a fun way for your kids to eat every day for the rest of their life. (A Healthier Kids 15 fun snack recipe guide is included in this plan).

Chapter 19

REMINDERS & TIPS ABOUT A HEALTHIER YOU

10 Tips for Detoxifying and Cleansing the Body

AHY TIP 1 – Pray and Meditate

- Daily prayer is the key to ask God for cleanliness to purify the body. Always start and end your day with prayer. Focus and meditate on healing the body from inside out. Seek God for deliverance for your healing. Whatever your circumstances are God has it all in control. Be faithful to the cause in knowing you are aiming to live a healthy lifestyle. Your body is God's temple. Therefore, treat it with kindness and nourish it with the plenty of good foods that The Lord has provided. Here are a few scriptures that will help with your daily detox and cleanse.

    o Suggested Scriptures:
      3 John 1:2, 1 Corinthians 6:19-20, 1 Corinthians 10:31, Romans 12:1-2, Genesis 1:29.

AHY TIP 2 – Reduce your Toxic Overload

- To reduce your toxic overload, eliminate process foods that causes the body to be sluggish, infected with diseases and weight gain. Reducing toxics from the body helps strengthens the body and allow healing to take place on the inside. The following will be helpful in reducing the toxic overload:

  - Transition to whole foods
  - Eliminate refine sugars, white flour, rice, breads, and white grains/pasta
  - Refined carbohydrates: donuts, pasta, cookies, chips
  - Alcohol: Wine, beer, liquor, spirits
  - Eliminate oils: Vegetable, Canola, Corn, Soy, and Cotton
  - No Cigarettes
  - No Dairy Products (Whole milk, cheese, etc).
  - Meats (Processed, fried, etc.)
  - Caffeine (Sodas and coffee)
  - Energy Drinks

AHY TIP 3 – Detoxifying and Cleansing the Body with Fruits and Vegetables

- Organic vegetables and fruit are great to buy and they are expensive. Organic products are free from pesticides and herbicides. If you can't buy organic, fresh fruits and vegetables would be good too. Prepare your daily smoothies, herbal teas, infused water, and meals with the fruits and vegetables.

  o Prepare smoothies with green leafy veggies (More greens then fruit)
  o Buy organic fruits and veggies if possible
  o Use frozen fruit for creamier smoothies
  o Wash fresh fruit, Ziploc bag them, and freeze. (If you don't want to freeze the fruit, wash them thorough before using)
  o Wash all veggies (Pre-wash veggies rinse). Don't wash the veggies before usage. Wash and freeze the veggies.

AHY TIP 4: Stop Using Toxic Chemicals in Your House

- Using aerosol cleaning products often invades the body causes toxin. To lower your chances from toxic overload with household chemicals. Make your household toxic chemical free:

- o Organic, all-purpose cleaner is great for kitchen counter tops, bathroom and kitchen sinks, toilet bowls – you name it.

- o Another great household detox: Instead of using Windex, use plain vinegar for cleaning glass and mirrors. (The mixture can be used in cleaning just about everything including makeup from the makeup brushes. After thoroughly cleaning with vinegar and water, use a lemon for freshness).

AHY TIP 5 – Drink Water, Drink Water, Drink Water

- Water is a great hydrated source to help flush the fat from your body. These few tips will get you started to make sure the body stays hydrated:

  - o Drink warm lemon water like a tea in the mornings. Lemon water can be consumed throughout the day.

  - o Drink water half your body weight in ounces daily. (Purified, distill or spring water).

  - o Drink infused water

AHY TIP 6 – Support the Liver Before and After the Cleanse

- The liver is essential for so many things, but most importantly, it is one of the most vital internal organ to **support weight loss.** Without the liver, and bile produced by the organ, we couldn't lose weight, no matter how much you exercise or eat sensible meals.

- The liver helps to create and process special enzymes called lipase that digest fats. Most of the toxins produced in the body are stored there and in our blood stream, which makes us, you know "fat". You must include the following to maintain a healthy liver:

  - Eat detoxifying foods daily to detox the liver naturally. (Lemon water does this automatically).

  - Having bowel movements frequently at least 2-3 times a day help keeps the liver free from toxins too.

AHY TIP 7 Detox Your Whole Body

- Detoxing your whole body is beneficial. Toxins can be pulled from the body like a magnet when you use the following methods:
  - Dry Body Brushing

- when you dry brush your body, you help remove your skin's dead cells, and are making room for new and

  fresh skin cells to grow. This helps the skin release toxins and can help reduce the toxic detox load on your liver and kidneys.

- Detox Bath

  - Soaking in a detox bath helps in relaxing the muscles, soreness, bloating, back pain, fever, allergies, constipation, relaxation, and more. (See *"Best Detox Bath Soak"* Chapter 14).

- Detox Foot Bath

  - Amplify your cleanse with this amazing detox foot bath to remove dead skin cells from the feet and draw out toxins.

AHY TIP 8: Relax, Relate, Retreat

- When you are doing a full-cleanse it is best to take it easy to give the body time to heal and adjust to the new way of absorbing nutrients. You will endure clarity, vitality, and serenity.

- Don't do any hard-core exercises because of the healing process. I suggest that you do brief walking and or non-strenuous exercises until after the full-cleanse.

- If you are doing the moderate cleanse you can do your daily routine exercise, but take in more proteins to burn the body fat. (Follow instructions on adding powder protein (plant based) to the smoothies. Eat bake, broiled, or grilled meats like fish and chicken no more than 4 to 6 ounces if you are trying to lose more weight.

- Lower your stress level and get to bed early. When your body rest and get the proper amount of sleep you lose weight.

AHY TIP 9: Detox Your Friends and May Be Family

- Just because you decided to work on you, there will be those who won't support you in making changes that you have desired for yourself.

- Be prepared to lose some friends and or family members who may have been lingering, clinging toxic invaders. Go ahead detox them too.

- You will feel better. Weight loss is no weight gain!".

- Join the online support group "A Healthier You w/Dr. V. Benson.

- You must strive to reach goal and keep it moving.

AHY TIP 10: Maintaining the weight loss

- Pray and meditate daily.
- Avoid eating foods that caused you to gain the weight in the first place.
- Restart the 10/14 once a month until you reach your ideal weight.
- Choose healthy meals, snacks, and drink smoothies to replace any meal.
- Exercise and take brief walks 3 times a week.
- Drink water for half your body weight.
- Drink lemon water every morning.
- Get at least 8 to 9 hours of sleep per day.
- Join A Healthier You VIP membership and A for continuous support and coaching.
- Join the Facebook page group.

  https://www.facebook.com/groups/AHealthierYouwDr.V.Benson/

"So whether you eat or drink, or whatever you do, do it all for the glory of God." 1 Corinthians 10:31 (NLT)

Prayer works! No matter what the circumstances are….

Chapter 20

UNLEASH OVER 100 SMOOTHIES: MIX & MATCH

Working on specific areas of the body will help you to continue to live healthy and happier. Some of the smoothies can be healthy to heal other areas in the body. Start your own regiment to gain optimal health with these tasty smoothies, Drink the smoothies 3 times or more per week. Mix and match these recipes or use as desired. To add sweetness to any of the smoothies add 1-2 packs of Stevia or raw honey to recipes that use these ingredients.

Directions: Blend all ingredients until smooth or creamy.

Beauty (Hair, Skin, and Nails Smoothies

Berry Berries

1 handful spinach

1 cup almond milk

1 banana

1 cup frozen mixed berries

1 tsp. ground flaxseeds

2 scoops hemp powder

Kiwi Mango Pineapple

1 cup frozen mango

4 kiwis, peeled

1 ½ cup frozen pineapple

4 mint leaves

Cranberry Pear Blast

2 red pears

½ cucumber

¾ cup frozen or fresh cranberries

¼ lemon peeled

½ tsp. ground ginger

Apple Green Grapefruit

1 grapefruit peeled

1 cored green apple

½ Cucumber

¼ cup swiss chard leaves

Super Skin Blast

2 handfuls baby spinach kale

½ lemon peeled

1/3 grapefruit peeled

1 cored red apple

1 celery stalk

1 tsps. ground ginger

½ cup cran-pomegranate juice (Ocean Spray Diet)

Anti-Aging Smoothies

Kale Honeydew Melon

1 handful kale

½ honey dew melon (rind removed)

1 cucumber

½ lemon peeled

Orange Strawberry Cream

½ cup plain Greek yogurt

¾ cup strawberry Greek yogurt

1 orange, deseeded and peeled

1 ½ cup frozen or fresh strawberries

Blueberry Orange

2 handfuls kale

1 cup blueberries

1 orange (deseeded and peeled)

1 tbsp. flaxseeds

1 handful Brazil nuts

Go Green

1 cup spinach

½ ripe banana

1 avocado (peeled and pit removed)

1 tbsp. sunflower seeds

½ cup lemon juice

1 cup unsweetened almond milk

Cool Pineapple Chia

1 cup coconut water

1 cup frozen pineapple chunks

½ cup frozen mango

1 tbsp. chia seeds

Creamy Cacao

1 cup frozen strawberries

1 banana

1 cup unsweetened almond or coconut milk

1 tbsp. cacao powder

Weight loss and Fat Buster Smoothies

Easy Green Lean Machine

1 cup spinach

1 cup fresh cilantro

2 stalks celery

5 leaves kale

½ cucumber

½ green apple

½ lemon peeled

½ tsp. ground ginger

Lime Sherbet

½ lime peeled, deseeded

½ cup unsweetened coconut milk

1cup low fat sherbet

½ cup raspberries

Apple Carrot

2 carrots

2 stalks celery

1 green apple

2 leaves kale

½ cup fresh parsley

Apple Cinnamon Cranberry

3 handful spinach

1 cup water

2 cored green apples

1 cup red seedless grapes or green seedless grapes

1½ cup frozen fresh cranberries (pitted cranberries if fresh)

2 celery stalks

1 bunch parsley

1 tsp. cinnamon

1 tsp. fresh turmeric (ground)

1 tbsps. flaxseeds (ground or mill)

1 stevia (Optional)

1 scoop protein (Optional)

Apple Ginger Mint

1 cucumber

½ cup water

10 fresh mint leaves

1 slice fresh ginger (washed and skinned)

2 cored green apples

Blueberry Fresh

½ cup plain Greek yogurt

½ cup water

1 cup frozen blueberries

Pomegranate Lime

1 cup Pom pomegranate juice

½ cucumber

¼ cup coconut water

1 lime peeled

Cashew Berry

2 handfuls spinach

½ cup frozen blueberries

½ cup strawberries

¼ cup raw cashews

2 tbsps. rolled oats

1 tbsp. flaxseeds (or ½ tbsp. flaxmeal)

1 ½ cup unsweetened almond milk

Grapefruit Apple Strawberry

1 handful spinach

1 handful kale

1 cored green apple

1 cup frozen strawberries

½ cup green grapes

¼ grapefruit

2 tbsps. flaxseeds (Grounded or milled)

Blueberry Spinach Coconut

1 handful spinach (Optional)

1 tbsp. coconut oil

½ cup frozen blueberries

1 tsp. nuts or seeds

½ cup unsweetened coconut milk

½ cup plain Greek yogurt

¼ cup rolled oats

1 stevia or to taste

Tropical Mango Banana

1 handful spinach

1 cup coconut water or unsweetened coconut milk

1 tbsp. coconut oil

½ cup frozen mango

1 banana

¼ cup pineapple juice

Bones and Joint Comfort (Arthritis, Rheumatoid, Osteoarthritis) Smoothies

Pineapple Mango

1 cup frozen pineapples or fresh pineapple

1 cup frozen mango

1 cucumber

1 lemon peeled

Citrus Ginger

½ cup broccoli florets

2 oranges peeled

1 grapefruit peeled, deseeded

1 zucchini

½ tsp. ground ginger

Apple Green Asparagus

4 spears asparagus

½ cup water

3 carrots

3 celery stalks

1 green apple

1 cup broccoli florets

1 cup fresh parsley

Spinach Pineapple

2 handfuls spinach

1 cup frozen pineapple

1 cored pear

1 cup parsley

½ grapefruit peeled

Hormone Balance Smoothies

Butternut Squash Super Smoothie

4 oz. butternut squash (baked)

1 pear cored chopped

1 tsp. cinnamon

3 tbsps. walnuts

1 tbsp. mesquite powder

1 tsp. extra virgin olive oil

1 cup water

1 cup ice

Bake the butter squash in extra virgin olive oil for 30 minutes. Cool for 15 minutes. Add to other ingredients to blend until smooth.

Almond Raspberry Spicy Sweet

1 handful spinach

4 oz. butternut squash (baked)

2 tbsp. coconut oil (1 tbsp. to coat the butter squash and 1 tbsp. to blend in smoothie)

½ cup almonds

1 cup coconut milk or almond milk

1tsp. cinnamon

1 tsp. vanilla extract

1tsp. grated or ground ginger

½ cup Medjool date

Bake the butter squash in 1 tbsp. coconut oil for 30 minutes. Cool for 15 minutes. Add to other ingredients to blend until smooth.

Avocado Green Cacao

2 handfuls baby spinach

1 cup water

¼ fresh frozen avocado (pitted and frozen until ready to use)

½ cup cashew nuts

1 tbsp. maca powder

2 tbsps. cacao powder

1 tbsp. hemp seeds

1 Stevia

Medjool Sunflower Butter

1 cup coconut milk

¼ cup water

2 Medjool date

1 tbsps. maca powder

¼ tsp. Himalayan pink salt

1 tsp. vanilla extract

1 scoop vanilla protein powder

1-2 tbsps. sunflower butter

1-2 tsps. raw honey

Royal Blueberry Honey

2 cups baby spinach

1 cup frozen blueberries

1 cup frozen mango

1 cup Greek coconut yogurt

2 tbsps. sesame seeds

1 tbsp. ground cardamom

1-2 tsps. raw honey

Spicy Almond Cardamom

1 cup almond milk

1 banana

1 tbsp. ground cardamom

2 tbsps. almond butter

1 tsp. raw honey

Constipation Smoothies

Apple Green Cabbage

¼ small green cabbage

1 cored green apple

¼ cup water

½ bulb fennel or 1 bag fennel tea (cooled)

½ lemon peeled

Prepare 1 bag of tea with 1 cup of water and steep 2-3 minutes before mixing with other ingredients.

Blueberry Pineapple Oats

2 cups water

1 cup steel cut oats

1 banana peeled

1 cup plain Greek yogurt

1 cup frozen blueberries

½ frozen pineapples

Soak the steel cut oats in 1 cup water for 10 minutes. Add to other ingredients with an additional cup of water.

Apple Hazelnut

1 cup hazelnut milk

1 cored red apple

1 kiwi peeled

1 cup kefir (Plain)

Peachy Grapes

1 ripe peach (Pitted)

1 cup frozen blueberries

½ cup red or green grapes

½ cup prunes

Allergies (colds, flu, headaches, sore throat, sinusitis) Smoothies

Headache Relief

1 cup water

1 cored green apple

1 cup cauliflower

1 cup broccoli florets

Apple Papaya Smoothie

2 handfuls kale

1 handful spinach

1 cored apple

1-2 cup water

1 cup frozen or fresh papaya

½ cup frozen or fresh strawberries

1 cup frozen or fresh peaches

2 tbsps. flaxseeds (ground or mill)

Tropical Lemon Orange Berry

2 handfuls spinach

1 cups water

1 cup seedless red grapes

1 cup frozen or fresh blueberries

1 orange peeled and deseeded

1 lemon peeled or ¼ cup lemon juice

1 lime peeled

1 tbsp. flaxseeds (ground or mill)

Spinach Kale Berry Smoothie

1 handful spinach

2 handfuls kale

1 cup water

1 banana peeled

1 bunch parsley

1 ½ cup frozen or fresh blueberries

1 ½ cup frozen or fresh blackberries

1 cup fresh red or black grapes

2 tbsps. flaxseeds (ground or mill)

Banana Pineapple Smoothie

2 handfuls spring mix greens

1 cup water

1 banana peeled

1 cup frozen pineapple chunks

1 cup fresh seedless red grapes

2 celery stalks chopped

2 slices ginger root (Washed and skinned) or 1 tsp. ground ginger

2 tbsps. flaxseeds (ground or mill)

Heart Healthy Smoothies

Broccoli Tomato

2 tomatoes

1 cup broccoli florets

1 carrot

1 stalk celery

½ fresh lemon peeled

1 clove, garlic

Avocado Kiwi

1 handful spring mixed power greens

1 cup orange juice

1 frozen pitted avocado (freeze fresh)

1 cup frozen peeled kiwi sliced

2 tbsps. flaxseeds or hemp seeds

Blueberry Avocado

1 cup coconut milk

1 cup strawberry Greek yogurt

1 ½ cup frozen blueberries

½ frozen pitted avocado (freeze fresh)

½ cup frozen strawberries

1 tsp. raw honey

2 tbsps. flaxseeds

Chocolate Blueberry Almond

1 ½ cup almond milk

1 cup steel oats

1 cup frozen blueberries

½ cup almonds

2 bars dark chocolate

1 tsp. raw honey

Healthy Kids Smoothies

Creamy Berry

1 ¼ cup whole milk or unsweetened almond or coconut milk

2 tbsps. lain Greek yogurt

1 tbsp. maple syrup

½ cup frozen or fresh blackberries

½ cup frozen or fresh blueberries

Cranberry Smooth

3 cups frozen cranberries

2 cups cranberry juice

1 ¼ cups plain Greek yogurt

2-3 tbsps. honey

Peach Raspberry

1 cup almond or coconut milk

1 ½ cup frozen raspberry

1 cup frozen mango

1 cup frozen sliced peaches

2 tsps. raw honey

Banana Walnut

1 banana

1 cup cooked oats

1 tsp. ground almond meal

1 cup unsweetened coconut milk

2 tbsps. plain Greek yogurt

2 tbsps. Chopped walnuts

1 pinch cinnamon

1 tsp. raw honey

Orange Apple Banana

1 cup orange juice

½ banana

½ apple

1 cup ice

Immunity Booster Smoothies

Green Berry Apple

1 cup collard greens (destemmed), Swiss chard or kale (Destemmed)

1 cup frozen or fresh blueberries

1 cored green apple

1 cucumber

½ fresh lemon peeled

Beet Orange

1 orange peeled

1 cup cooked beet, (chopped)

5 tbsps. plain Greek yogurt

2/3 cup water

Strawberry Colada

4 cups frozen or fresh strawberries

½ cup coconut cream

2 ½ cups frozen pineapples

Green Apple Spinach Walnut

2 handfuls spinach

1 Persian cucumber

1 cored green apple

1 bag Matcha maker green tea (Make tea with 1 cup of water)

½ fresh squeezed lemon

1 tsp. ginger

Steep tea for 2-3 minutes and cool. Add tea into other ingredients and blend until smoothie.

Edema (Bloating and Swelling) Smoothies

Pineapple Cranberry Kale

1 cup kale

1 cup parsley

1 celery stalk

1 cucumber

1 cup frozen or fresh pineapples

1 cup frozen or fresh cranberries (Pitted)

Banana Strawberry Orange

1 handful spinach

½ cup water

1 banana

1 cup strawberries

1 squeezed orange or ¼ cup unsweetened orange juice

½ cup of walnuts

Carrot Apple Cucumber

1 cored apple

¼ cup water

1 carrot

½ cucumber

Pineapple Carrot

2 carrots

½ cup frozen pineapples

1 cup pineapple juice (100%)

Mango Melon

½ cantaloupe melon (deseeded)

2½ cups frozen mango

2 oranges peeled

Apple Celery

1 cored apple

2 celery stalks

1 cup unsweetened coconut milk

1 stevia

Anti-Stress (Calmness, Anxiety Relief) Smoothies

Raspberry Walnut

1 banana

1 cup frozen or fresh raspberry

1 cup unsweetened coconut milk

1 tbsp. flaxseed

½ cup walnuts

Tropical Pineapple Blueberry Lime

1 cup unsweetened coconut milk

1 cup frozen pineapples

1 cup frozen blueberries

½ cup lime (100%) juice

1 tbsp. bee pollen

Avocado Blueberry Mango

1 cup unsweetened coconut milk

1 cup frozen or fresh blueberries

1 cup frozen or fresh mango

½ cup almonds

1 tsp. cinnamon

1 handful pecans (Optional)

Banana Pineapple Walnut

1 cup unsweetened coconut milk

1 banana peeled

1 cup frozen or fresh pineapple

½ cup walnuts

Cran-Pomegranate Berry

1 handful kale

1 frozen banana

½ cup frozen mixed berries

1 cup frozen blueberries

½ cup cran-pomegranate (Ocean Spray 100% Juice)

1 tbsp. hemp seed

1 tbsp. flaxseeds (Grounded or milled)

Carrot Banana Mango

2 carrots

1 banana

1 cup frozen pineapple

1 cup frozen mango

½ cup walnuts

Spinach Almond

1 handful spinach

1 cup unsweetened almond milk

1 tbsp. coconut oil

1 banana peeled

1 cup frozen mango

½ cup walnuts

Avocado Greek Yogurt

1 cup Greek yogurt

1 cup unsweetened almond milk

1 avocado (Pitted)

1 carrot

½ cup walnuts

1 tsp. cinnamon

1 tsp. nutmeg

Nectarine Orange

1 cup c or almond milk

5 nectarines (pitted)

1 squeezed orange (deseeded)

1 cup frozen strawberries

1 avocado (pitted)

½ cup vanilla bean powder

Cashew Banana Kiwi

1 handful kale

1 cup water

1 banana peeled

2 kiwis peeled

1 cup frozen pineapple

¼ cup cashews

Blueberry Spinach

1 handful spinach

1 cup frozen blueberries

¼ avocado

1 tsp. ginger grounded

1tsp. chia seeds

1 cup coconut water

Diabetes Control Smoothies

Pineapple-Strawberry Green Smoothie

2 handfuls kale

½ cup fresh parsley

2 cups frozen or fresh pineapple

1 cups whole or frozen strawberries

1 banana peeled

1 tbsp. hemp seeds

Apple Cinnamon

1 cored Apple

1 banana peeled

1 carrot

1 celery stalk

1 sweet potato (baked)

1 lemon (peeled and deseeded)

1 tsp. of cinnamon powder

1/2 tsp. of cayenne pepper

1 cup of fresh water

Kale Apple Green Pear

2 handfuls kale (remove stems)

1 coconut milk

1 cored green apple

1 fresh frozen lime (peeled, deseeded, and frozen)

1 cored pear

½ cup mint leaves

2 tbsps. flaxseeds

1 tsp. raw honey

Energizer Wake-up Morning, Afternoon or Evening Smoothies

Sun-Up Pineapple Banana

1 frozen banana

1 cup frozen pineapple

1 cup frozen mango

½ cup plain Greek yogurt

½ cup orange

1 tsp. grated ginger or 1tsp. ground ginger

Banana Pineapple Lime

2 bananas peeled

1 cup frozen pineapple

½ lime, Peeled or ½ cup lime Juice

Banana Berry Cherry

1 frozen banana

1 cup frozen dark red cherries

1 cup frozen blueberries

1 cup water

Get-up Orange

1 cup plain Greek yogurt

1 cup frozen peaches

1 cup frozen peeled oranges

½ cup small baby carrots

Galla Melon Smoothie

½ cup pineapple juice (100%)

1 orange (peeled and deseeded)

¼ cup Galla melon (cut in chunks)

1 cup frozen pineapple chunks

Orange Tomato

1 orange (peeled and deseeded)

1 cup tomato juice

1 cucumber

Carrot Ginger

1 cup carrots

½ cup water

4 tomatoes skinned

1 tbsp. lemon juice

$^{1/3}$ cup fresh parsley

1tbsp. ground ginger

Carrot Tomato Pepper

1 cup carrot juice

1 cup tomato juice

2 large red peppers (deseeded and chopped)

1 tbsp. lemon juice

1 tsp. freshly grounded black pepper (Optional topping)

Coconut Banana Greens

1-2 cups unsweetened coconut milk or almond milk or (mixed brand)

2 handfuls kale

2 handfuls spinach

½ avocado

2 frozen bananas

1 tsp. fresh or grounded ginger

½ tsp. chia or flaxseeds

½ tsp. raw honey

1 tsp. hemp powder

2 scoops plant base protein

Tomato Hot Pepper

2 cups tomato juice or 2 fresh tomatoes

1 small red Chile (deseeded and chopped)

1 scallion (chopped)

Strawberry Cherry Blast

1 cup water

1 cup frozen strawberries

1 cup frozen cherries

1 orange (deseeded)

1tbsp. chia seeds

1 tsp. agave or 1 Stevia

Spinach Matcha

1 handful kale or spinach

1 cup almond milk

1 banana

1 tbsp. coconut oil

1-2 tsp. matcha green tea powder

¼ tsp. cinnamon

¼ tsp. almond extract (optional)

Performance Endurance Smoothies

Kiwi Strawberry Apple

1 cup kale

½ cup water

2 cored apples

2 kiwis peeled

½ cup frozen strawberries

½ fresh lime peeled

Orange Strawberry Cream

½ cup plain Greek yogurt

1 cup almond or coconut milk

¾ cup strawberry yogurt

½ orange (peeled and deseeded)

1½ cup frozen or fresh strawberries

Green Apple

1 handful spinach or kale

1 tsp. chia seed

¼ cup water

1 green apple

10 mint leaves

½ cup apple juice (100 %)

Banana Almond Butter

1 cup coconut milk

¼ cup water

1 banana

2 tsp. almond butter

1 scoop whey protein

Pineapple Green Grapes

1 cup almond milk

¼ cup water

1 cup frozen grapes

1 cup frozen pineapple chunks

1 scoop Whey Protein

Banana Mango

1 cup coconut milk

2 tbsp. raw coconut butter

1 frozen banana

1 cup frozen mango

2 tbsp. flaxseeds

1 scoop whey protein

Honey Strawberry

1 banana peeled

1 cup frozen or fresh strawberries

1 cup frozen or fresh peaches

2 tbsps. raw honey

1 cup apple juice (100%)

Pineapple Raspberry Protein Shake

2 handfuls spinach

1 -11oz. Premier vanilla protein shake

1 cup frozen or fresh pineapples

1 cup frozen or fresh raspberries

Blackberry Banana

2 handfuls baby spinach

1 cup frozen blackberries

½ cup frozen raspberries

1 banana peeled

½ fresh avocado

1/3 cup fresh mint leaves

½ cup water

½ cup raw almonds

Apple Banana Mint (Post Workout)

1 cup milk or plain Greek yogurt

1 cored apple

1 banana

5-6 mint leaves

1-2 tsp. raw honey

pinch sea salt

Chronic Illnesses & Other Disorder Smoothies

(pancreatitis, fibromyalgia, diabetes, autism, cancer prevention, hypertension, high cholesterol, fibroids, impotence, Alzheimer, digestive disorders and other chronic illness).

Cucumber Ginger

1 cucumber

1 beet

½ cup water

1 fresh lemon peeled

2 slices ginger Root (washed and skinned)

½ jalapeno pepper

Super Carrot Blast

1 handful Bok Choy

1 handful kale

1 cup water

1 cord green apple

4 carrots

2 slices ginger root (washed and skinned)

Kiwi Peach Patch

2 handfuls spinach or Swiss chard

3 kiwis

1 ½ cup frozen peaches

1 avocado (pitted and diced)

2 tbsps. lime juice

1 ½ cup pineapple juice

Apple Carrot Zest

2 cored green apples

¼ cucumber

½ cup water

1 tsp. ground ginger

Peachy Me

1½ handfuls spinach

½ cup water

1 cup frozen or fresh peaches

3 mint leaves

Pear Spinach

2 cups fresh spinach

2 cucumbers

½ cup water

1 cores pear

½ fresh lemon peeled

1 slice fresh ginger root (Washed and skinned)

Super Red

1 red beet

2 red pears

½ cup red grapes

1½ cups frozen or fresh raspberries

1 cup frozen or fresh strawberries

½ cucumber

Red Sunset Berry

1 cup frozen strawberries

½ cup frozen dark red cherries

1 orange (Deseeded and peeled)

½ fresh lime peeled

Spinach Red Blast

1 handful spinach

½ cup water

1 carrot

½ cucumber

1 plum (pitted)

½ cup frozen strawberries

¼ cup frozen dark red cherries

Papaya Banana

1 papaya

1 fresh lime peeled

1 banana peeled

2 oranges (deseeded and peeled)

¼ tsp. grounded ginger

Tropical Papaya Pineapple

1 cup frozen papaya

½ cup frozen pineapple

2/3 cup unsweetened coconut or almond milk

1½ cup plain Greek yogurt

Blueberry Red Cabbage

¼ red cabbage

1 hand kale

1 hand Swiss chard

1 celery stalk

1 cup alkaline water

1 cup frozen blueberries

1 cup frozen blackberries

1 cup frozen strawberries

1 tsp. turmeric

Avocado Mango Green

2 handfuls spring mixed greens

½ cup water

½ cup mango

1 avocado (pitted

1 banana

½ lemon lime (peeled)

Kale Banana Almond

¾ cup kale (remove stem)

1 small frozen banana

¾ cup unsweetened almond milk

1 tsp. almond butter

1/8 tsp. cinnamon

1/8 tsp. nutmeg

1/8 tsp. ginger

Cherry Almond

1 cup unsweetened almond milk

1 cup cherries

1 tbsp. almond butter

1 tsp. vanilla extract

1 tsp. almond extract

2 tbsps. Flaxseeds (ground or milled)

Chapter 21

MY 10/14 FIT & SMOOTHIE JOURNEY

Start Date: _____   End Date: _____

Starting Weight: _____   Ending Weight: _____

Day 1:

_____

_____

_____

_____

_____

Day 2:

_____

_____

_____

_____

_____

Day 3:

_____

_____

_____

_____

_____

Day 4:

_____

_____

_____

_____

Day 5:

_____

_____

_____

_____

Day 6:

_____

_____

_____

_____

_____

Day 7:

_____

_____

_____

_____

_____

Day 8:

_____

_____

_____

_____

_____

Day 9:

_____

_____

_____

_____

_____

Day 10:

_____

_____

_____

_____

_____

Day 11:

_____

_____

_____

_____

Day 12:

_____

_____

_____

_____

Day 13:

_____

Day 14:

My Daily Prayer:

My 5- Day Smoothie Recipes: More Greens/Less Fruit

Recipe 1:

Recipe 2:

Recipe 3:

Recipe 4:

Recipe 5:

About the Author

Dr. Vickie Benson is a native of Tuskegee, Alabama. She is a graduate of Alabama State University where she received multiple degrees; Bachelor of Science in Biology, Masters of Education in Biology Education, Masters of Education in Educational Administration P-12 and an Education Specialist in Educational Administration P-12. Dr. Benson received her doctorate from Argosy University in Educational Leadership K-12. She also graduated from the University of Alabama at Birmingham where she received training and a certificate in Medical Assistant.

As a 20-year veteran science teacher and educational coach, Dr. Benson's passion for educating others about wellness and maintenance for a healthy lifestyle will help others to move in the same direction to become healthy. Her goal is to publish her second book on healthy eating and teacher effectiveness in the classroom. Teachers lose interest due to job anxiety and stress which leads to chronic illnesses such as hypertension and diabetes. She believes, *"When teachers are healthy, they are effective in their craft and students achieve more"*.

With detoxing and cleansing, Dr. Benson has regained clarity, vitality, and serenity. She has a total new outlook on life and dare not to miss taking in her smoothies daily. The outcome from detoxing and cleansing were very positive. Detoxing and cleansing allowed her to unleash an empowerment of changes for a lifetime. While writing this book, Dr. Benson believed that it is a blessing from God to utilize what He has given her to share and educate others on how to become healthy through a weight loss plan called *"10/14 Fit & Smoothie Cleanse"*. She also designed *"A Healthier You Six Tier Plan"* consisting of 6 optimal eating healthy plans that will possibly help the body in healing various chronic illnesses, disorders, revert bad eating habits to good eating habits, and weight loss.

Dr. Benson is the founder of educational solutions consultants which focuses on providing academic consultations for high school/college students for transition and college entrance. Her new project focus, *"Healthy Educators Are Effective Educators: Love Thy Teaching Without the Stress and Anxiety"*. She is a God-fearing woman and praises God for her good health and healing through detoxing and cleansing. In hope, she, in return wants to inspire and motivate others to become healthier through detoxing and cleansing.

Dr. Benson loves to cook for her family and design great recipes. She encourages her family daily to be more health conscious. Her greatest past time is spending special occasions with her loving family and taking pictures of their moments together to post on Facebook, if she is not whipping up healthy smoothies. She is a devoted mother to Nikeyta, grandma Nana to her handsome grandson Landon, and a loving wife to Lee.